U0221584

Coronary Artery Fistula

Adviser
Junbo Ge

Editors
**Jufang Chi, Hangyuan Guo,
Xiaojie Xie, Shitian Guo**

Secretaries
**Jueting Wei, Mingliao Zhu,
Hanlin Zhang, Fang Wang**

ZHEJIANG UNIVERSITY PRESS
浙江大学出版社
·杭州·

图书在版编目（CIP）数据

冠状动脉瘘 = Coronary Artery Fistula：英文 /
池菊芳等编. —杭州：浙江大学出版社，2023.6
ISBN 978-7-308-23916-5

Ⅰ.①冠… Ⅱ.①池… Ⅲ.①冠状血管－动脉疾病－
诊疗－英文 Ⅳ.①R543.3

中国国家版本馆 CIP 数据核字（2023）第 103657 号

冠状动脉瘘

池菊芳　郭航远
谢小洁　郭诗天　　编

责任编辑　余健波
责任校对　何　瑜
封面设计　周　灵
出版发行　浙江大学出版社
　　　　　　（杭州市天目山路 148 号　邮政编码 310007）
　　　　　　（网址：http://www.zjupress.com）
排　　版　杭州好友排版工作室
印　　刷　杭州宏雅印刷有限公司
开　　本　710mm×1000mm　1/16
印　　张　21.5
字　　数　532 千
版 印 次　2023 年 6 月第 1 版　2023 年 6 月第 1 次印刷
书　　号　ISBN 978-7-308-23916-5
定　　价　138.00 元

Abbreviation

ACA—anomalous coronary arteries;

ACAOS—anomalous origin of a coronary artery from the opposite sinus;

ACAVF—aortocoronary arteriovenous fistula;

ACS—acute coronary syndrome;

ALCAPA—anomalous origin of the LCA from PA;

AMB—acute marginal branch;

AMI—acute myocardial infarction;

AN/An—coronary artery aneurysm;

AO—aorta;

AsAo—ascending aorta;

ASD—atrial septal defect;

AVP—Amplatzer vascular plug;

Bp—blood pressure;

CAA—coronary artery anomalies;

CABG—coronary artery bypass grafting;

CAD—coronary atherosclerotic disease;

CAF—coronary artery fistula;

CAP—coronary artery perforation;

CAPF—coronary artery-pulmonary fistula;

CAVF—coronary arteriovenous fistula;

CBF—coronary-bronchial artery fistula;

CCF—coronary-cameral fistula;

CDE—color Doppler echocardiography;

CDFI—color Doppler flow imaging;

CHD—congenital heart diseases;

CHF—congestive heart failure;

CPB—cardiopulmonary bypass;

CPDA—coronary posterior descending artery;

CS—coronary sinus;

CTA—computed topography angiography;

CT—computed tomographic;

CTO—chronic total occlusions;

CXR—chest X-ray;

D1/D—first diagonal branch;

DCM—dilated cardiomyopathy;

ECG—electrocardiography;

Echo—echocardiography;

HL—high lateral branch;

HOCM—hypertrophic obstructive cardiomyopathy;

ICA—invasive coronary angiography;

IE—infective endocarditis;

IVS—interventricular septum;

IVUS—intravascular ultrasound;

LAA—left atrial appendage;

LAD—left anterior descending artery;

LA—left atrial;

LCA—left coronary artery;

LCX—left circumflex branch;

LGE—late gadolinium enhancement;

LM/LMCA—left main coronary artery;

LPV—left pulmonary vein;

LSV—left sinus of Valsalva;

LV—left ventricular;

MDT—multidisciplinary team;

MIS—minimally invasive surgery;

MMF—multiple micro-fistula;

MPA—main pulmonary artery;

N-proBNP—N-terminal pro-B-type natriuretic peptide;

MR—magnetic resonance imaging;

MSCT/MDCT—multislice/multidetector computed tomography;

NSTEMI—non-ST elevation myocardial infarction;

OM—obtuse marginal branch;

OMT—optimal medical treatment;

PA—pulmonary artery;

PCI—percutaneous coronary intervention;

PDA—patent ductus arteriosus;

PL—posterolateral branch;

PLSVC—persistent left superior vena cava;

RA—right atrial;

RCA—right coronary artery;

RPA—right pulmonary artery;

RSCA—right subclavian artery;

RSV—right sinus of Valsalva;

RV—right ventricular;

SCA—single coronary artery;

SCD—sudden cardiac death;

SVCS—superior vena cava syndrome;

SVC—superior vena cava;

TCC—transcatheter closure;

TEE—transesophageal echocardiography;

TMT—treadmill test;

TOF—tetralogy of Fallot;

TTE—transthoracic echocardiography;

TV—tricuspid valve;

VSD—ventricular septal defect;

VT—ventricular tachyarrhythmia.

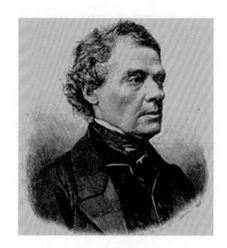

Josef Hyrtl

Austrian Anatomist

(1810—1894)

Coronary artery fistula (CAF) is a rare defect and aberrant connection between coronary arteries and other adjacent structures. They are usually small but can lead to several life-threatening complications, especially the large fistula. As a result, appropriate diagnosis with invasive coronary angiography (ICA) and treatment with transcatheter catheterization or surgical closure is necessary.

CAF can be divided into two categories: coronary-cameral fistula (CCF) and coronary arteriovenous fistula (CAVF), congenital and acquired. The most common cause of CAF is abnormal embryogenesis, and other important causes include: trauma (stab injury or gunshot), invasive procedures (intervention, coronary artery bypass grafting, valve replacement, device implantation, or endomyocardial biopsy), and cardiac surgery (septal myomectomy).

Although there are more and more studies regarding the prevalence of CAF in the general population, the prevalence of CAF was around 0.05% to 0.25%, as imaged by standard ICA. However, with the increasing use of CT angiography (CTA), this prevalence was found to be 0.9% – 1.0%, and the most common malformation was coronary artery-PA fistula. CAF is diagnosable at any age. However, diagnosis is usually made in early childhood, when an asymptomatic child or child with symptoms of congestive heart failure (CHF) presents with a heart murmur. No gender or race predilection has been noted in patients with CAF.

CAF can lead to several cardiopulmonary functional abnormalities. The severity of the presenting symptoms depends on the origin, drainage site and length of the fistula, as well as the shunt volume. The most common origin is RCA, and the most common drainage sites (from most common to least common) are the right ventricle (RV), right atrium (RA), and pulmonary artery (PA). However, the newer studies have shown that the most common fistula is between the left main artery (LM) or the left anterior descending artery (LAD) and PA.

Several studies have shown that CAF has thicker tunica intima and media with tightly packed smooth muscle cells. The anomalous arteries stained positive for alpha-smooth muscle actin (SMA), calponin, and desmin. The endothelium was found to be CD34 positive. Often, the anomalies would be accompanied by aneurysmal dilation at the neck of the aberrant coronary artery.

Generally speaking, CAF remains asymptomatic for 20 or so years. However, once the CAF starts to become hemodynamically significant, signs and symptoms can develop. Ischemia of the myocardium distal to the CAF may occur in some cases, referred to as the steal phenomenon. This situation results in angina syndrome, particularly in conditions associated with increased myocardial oxygen demand during infant feeding or exercises in adults. In infants, the symptoms manifest as diaphoresis, irritability, tachycardia, and tachypnea, and older adults with CHF present with dyspnea, palpitations, fatigue, orthopnea, paroxysmal nocturnal dyspnea, and lower limb swelling.

Clinical examination findings include: signs of CHF or cardiac tamponade, collapsing pulse, wide pulse pressure, diffuse apex beat, palpable third heart sound (S3), loud continuous murmur on auscultation, and atrial/ventricular arrhythmia.

Initial diagnostic exams could include laboratory tests (cardiac enzymes and B-type natriuretic peptide), chest X-ray, and electrocardiography

(ECG). Although these modalities do not yield a sufficient diagnosis, they help uncover some complications. Other valuable diagnostic methods of diagnosis of CAF include transthoracic echocardiography (TTE), color Doppler echocardiography (CDE), transesophageal Echo (TEE), MR/CT angiography (CTA), nuclear imaging, cardiac catheterization, and ICA. Not only is coronary CTA noninvasive, but it is also able to detect CAF at a higher rate as compared to standard ICA.

The differential diagnosis of CAF includes the followings: pulmonary arteriovenous malformation, intrathoracic systemic fistula, congenital systemic fistula to the pulmonary vein, ruptured aneurysm of coronary sinus (CS), patent ductus arteriosus (PDA), acute myocardial ischemia, CHF, arrhythmia, cardiac tamponade, and vasculitides such as Takayasu arteritis or Kawasaki disease.

Treatment and further management are only indicated in patients with the followings: hemodynamically significant left-right shunt, CHF with either LV volume overload or dysfunction, and myocardial ischemia. Although the surgical repair was once considered a treatment for CAF, with a higher level of fistula recurrence, recently, transcatheter closure (TCC) has become the gold standard technique. Patients are then given antiplatelet therapy and, in some cases, anticoagulants, for the first 6 months after cardiac catheterization.

The majority of presentations of patients with CAF are usually secondary to its complications. The followings are the list of complications that could be caused by CAF: ischemia due to stealing syndrome, CHF, thrombosis/embolism, arrhythmia, rupture, and endocarditis/endarteritis. Complications of TCC include coronary artery spasm, ventricular arrhythmia, coronary artery perforation or dissection, and myocardial ischemia from coronary artery thrombosis or improper positioning of occlusive devices. Complications of surgical closure include cardiac ischemia or AMI, and recurrence of CAF.

Life expectancy for patients with CAF is normal. Results of many studies indicate that both transcatheter and surgical approaches are associated with a good prognosis. In adults, some patients may remain asymptomatic for their entire lives if the fistula is not hemodynamically significant. In other patients with ensuing complications, an immediate reversal of the complication (surgery or TCC) is necessary to decrease morbidity. Although recurrence of the CAF is rare, surgery is known to increase the risk of recurrence compared with TCC. The need for additional surgery to treat recurrent CAF only presents in 4% of patients.

Patient education is highly important. The patients should receive education about the disease, management options, and possible complications associated with CAF and its treatment. They need to understand the importance of follow-up after discharge from the hospital. Once diagnosed, it is important to tell patients that CAF can become symptomatic after 2 decades or less, including chest pain, exertional dyspnea, palpitation and other cardiopulmonary symptoms. They should be demanded to undergo regular follow-up with Echo, Chest X-ray, ECG, and CTA or ICA.

The diagnosis and management of CAF are highly dependent on an effective interprofessional or multidisciplinary team (MDT). In pediatric patients, it is essential for nursing staff to monitor the vital signs of the neonate/infant and check for any clues of tachypnea or tachycardia. Neonatologists and pediatricians are first-line to differentiate and diagnose any murmurs of infant patients, therefore referring these patients to a pediatric cardiologists.

In adult patients, hospitalists and cardiologists should work together to appropriately diagnose and evaluate patients with CAF. Depending on the treatment selected, interventional cardiologists should be consulted to perform percutaneous TCC, or a cardiothoracic surgery service team should be consulted for surgical repair of the fistula. The nursing staff will coordinate the work of different team members and provide direct and considerate care by checking vital signs, administering medications, and attending to patients' needs.

Take-home messages

—CAF is a rare entity, and clinically relevant CAF is even rarer.

—In adults, the diagnosis is usually made incidentally by ICA or CTA, in the course of a routine investigation for causes of chest pain or CHF.

—Clinical presentation and severity of symptoms depend on the origin, insertion site, size, and length of the fistula, as well as the shunt volume.

—Management should be supported by an established definite mechanistic correlation of symptoms and/or functional abnormalities of the heart with the anatomical characteristics and magnitude of the flow through CAF. Functional assessment by right heart catheterization and ischemia assessment may be needed to establish this correlation.

—After a thorough assessment, patients with the following conditions should be considered for intervention: hemodynamically significant left-right shunt with right chamber enlargement or dysfunction and/or pulmonary hypertension, CHF with LV volume overload or LV dysfunction, or myocardial ischemia.

—Percutaneous treatment is the preferred therapy, however, there is high variability in anatomy, making device choice and complete closure challenging, and not all anatomies are suited for TCC.

—No specific dedicated device exists for this indication; devices from the occluder portfolio, coils, or covered stents are usually used according to the morphologic characteristics of CAF.

—Safety and efficacy are still a concern, given the overall low volume and the challenging technical demands of these cases.

—As with other heart conditions, surgery should be considered when there are other indications for surgery, or when TCC is not technically feasible or safe.

—Ligation of small incidental CAF may be considered at the time of surgery for other indications, according to the estimated risk of progression to a significant hemodynamic fistula, based on the size and length of the fistula, the vessels or chamber involved, and the patient's age.

—Treatment should be restricted to highly experienced centers and operators, in order to maximize success and safety.

CONTENTS

Preface

Postscript

Chapter I Overview

Highlights

- CAF is a rare congenital or acquired epicardial coronary connection with a cardiac chamber or great vessel.

- CAF is usually diagnosed incidentally.

- CAF can present with various anatomic configurations and clinical syndromes.

- The majority of CAF are asymptomatic.

- CAF can cause CHF, myocardial ischemia, and arrhythmia.

- Large or symptomatic CAF need intervention. Single, proximal, and non-tortuous CAF can be treated percutaneously; tortuous, distal, and multiple CAF need surgical closure.

- Closure may be an effective treatment for carefully selected symptomatic CAF.

- Large registries are needed to understand the natural history of various CAF.

As the aorta exits LV, 2 coronary arteries originate from its root to supply the muscles and tissues of the heart. The left coronary artery (LCA) originates from the left aortic sinus, while the right coronary artery (RCA) originates from the right aortic sinus. As the RCA descends a sinoatrial nodal, obtuse marginal branch (OM), and posterior interventricular, the LCA gives an anterior interventricular branch and a circumflex branch (Figure 1-1).

1. Coronary artery anomalies (CAA)

CAA is an uncommon finding but can be of significant clinical importance in a small number of individuals. Clinical presentation depends

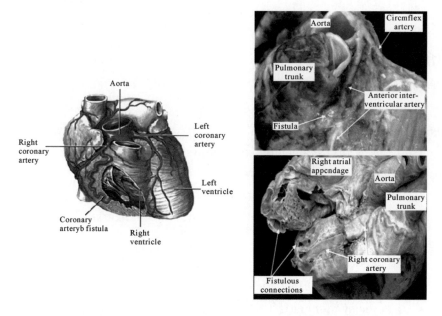

Figure 1-1 Model and autopsy findings of coronary artery and fistula.

on the specific anomaly. Most CAA are benign and clinically insignificant; however, some anomalies are potentially significant and can lead to CHF and even death. Their clinical significance is derived from the possibility of myocardial ischemia, ventricular tachycardia (VT), and other potential complications of sudden cardiac death (SCD). In asymptomatic, young, and athletic individuals, up to 15% of cases of SCD associated with increased physical activities were the result of an anomalous coronary artery origin.

Classification criteria for CAA have been extensively discussed in the literature. Some authors prefer to categorize CAA only as "major", "severe", "important", or "hemodynamically significant" anomalies versus "minor" ones. CAA is a group of congenital conditions characterized by abnormal origin or course of any of the 3 main epicardial coronary arteries. Such a scheme should include 2 basic steps: (a) The normal coronary anatomy (Table 1-1) should be described in terms of qualitative criteria, and (b) once the normal features have been excluded, the remaining features should be considered to define abnormality and used to generate a classification order

(Figures 1-2, 1-3).

Table 1-1   Normal features of the coronary anatomy in humans

Feature	Range
No. of ostia	2 to 4
Location	right and left anterior sinus (upper midsection)
Proximal orientation	45°– 90° off the aortic wall
Proximal common stem or trunk	only left (LAD and LCX)
Proximal course	direct, from ostium to destination
Mid-course	extramural (subepicardial)
Branches	adequate for the dependent myocardium
Essential territories	RCA (RV free wall), LAD (anteroseptal), or OM (LV free wall)
Termination	capillary bed

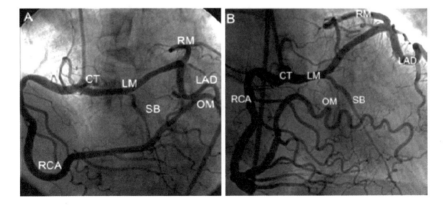

Figure 1-2   Angiograms from a 52-year-old man, in the left anterior oblique cranial (A) and right anterior oblique (B) projections. The patient had atypical chest pain and borderline nuclear stress test results. In these views, the whole coronary system is visualized from a single ostium located at the right sinus. This is a case of a clinically benign single coronary artery, which should more properly be called single coronary ostium because all the coronary arteries are present. However, they are anomalous in their origin and course.

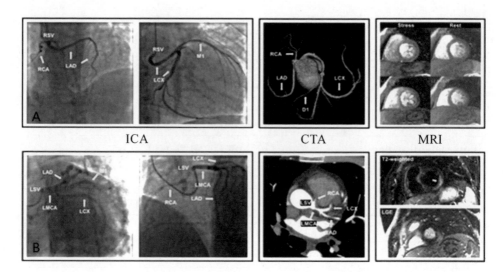

Figure 1-3 Real-life examples of CAA as unexpected findings. A: A 44-year-old man with typical chest pain, ICA showed no significant coronary stenosis; instead, an unexpected abnormality was observed: LAD originated from the right aortic sinus, sharing the same ostium with RCA, and LCX emerged from the right aortic sinus but from a separate and higher ostium. CTA showed a subpulmonic and a retroaortic course of LAD and LCX, respectively. MR demonstrated diffuse subendocardial inducible ischemia not matching any specific coronary supplied territory. The patient was treated conservatively; B: A 42-year-old man with sudden onset of oppressive chest pain and no coronary occlusion or stenosis were found, but RCA had an abnormal origin from the left aortic sinus. At CTA, RCA had an initial interatrial course, with a slight lumen reduction that was more evident during systole. Cardiac MR was performed to assess the presence and extent of myocardial necrosis but rather revealed morphological findings suggestive of acute myocarditis.

According to the classification principle of Schlesinger, not according to the site of origin or proximal course, the distribution of coronary artery was divided into 3 types: right dominant type; balanced type; left dominant type (Table 1-2 and Figure 1-4). CAA is most often identified as unexpected findings at Echo or ICA or coronary CTA during the diagnostic workup of ischemic heart disease. First-level functional tests (i. e. exercise ECG, stress Echo, or nuclear imaging) may then be proposed to assess the presence of CAA-related myocardial ischemia. However, second-level tests [such as coronary CTA, single-photon emission computed tomography (SPECT), or cardiac MRI] may be more accurate in this clinical context by establishing the potential matching between the CAA and the ischemic territories (Figures 1-5, 1-6).

Table 1-2   Simplified nomenclature of CAA

Type of anomaly	Variant	Subvariant
Anomalies of origin	Anomalous pulmonary origin of coronary artery	Origin of LM from PA Origin of RCA from PA Origin of LCX from PA Origin of LCA and RCA from PA
	Anomalous aortic origin of coronary artery	Origin of LM from the right aortic sinus Origin of RCA from the left aortic sinus Origin of LAD from the right aortic sinus Origin of LAD from RCA Origin of LCX from the right aortic sinus Origin of LCX from RCA Single coronary artery Inverted coronary arteries Others
	Congenital atresia of LM	
Anomalies of course	Myocardial (or coronary) bridging	Symptomatic/Asymptomatic
	Coronary artery aneurysm (AN)	Congenital/Acquired
Anomalies of termination	Coronary arteriovenous fistula	Congenital/Acquired
	Coronary stenosis	Congenital/Acquired

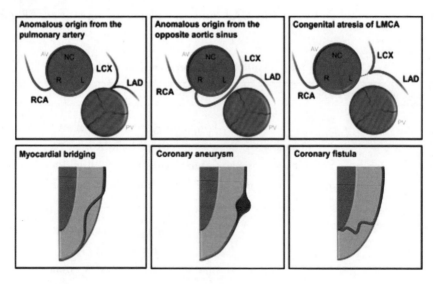

Figure 1-4 Schematic representation of the major types of CAA. AV: Aortic valve; L: Left coronary sinus; NC: Noncoronary sinus; PV: Pulmonary valve; R: Right coronary sinus.

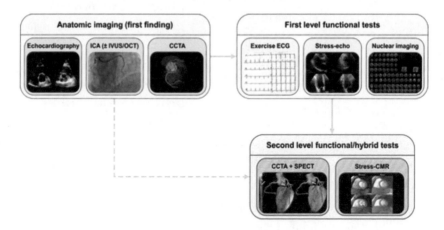

Figure 1-5 Inspection process of CAF.

2. Definition of CAF

The coronary artery directly communicates with the cardiac cavity or large vessel resembling a systemic or pulmonary circulation, without passing through the capillary network (Figure 1-6), and its pathophysiological changes are the same, which can be collectively referred to as CAVF or CAF.

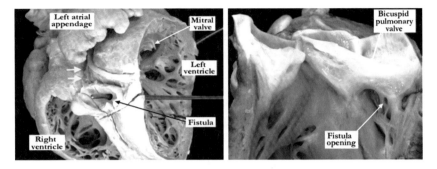

Figure 1-6   Autopsy findings of CAF.

CAF is a rare anomaly of the coronary arteries which results from an abnormal connection between a coronary artery with a cardiac chamber or vessel. The coronary steal phenomenon can lead to functional ischemia of the myocardium. The condition has been described extensively. However, the modalities for diagnosing this condition continue to advance.

The definitions offered by Chiu CZ and Gupta-Malhotra M were applied.

—Congenital CCF: Small or large, single or multiple fistulous connections originating from any of the coronary arteries and terminating into any of the cardiac chambers (RA, RV, LA, and LV).

—Solitary macro-fistula: These are single or multiple, small (< 1.5 mm) or large fistulas (> 1.5 mm), originating mainly from the proximal segment of coronary artery and entering into the cardiac chamber.

—Coronary artery-left ventricular multiple micro-fistula (MMF): These are multiple small channels originating from the mid or distal part of one or more coronary arteries draining more often into the left than the right ventricular cavity.

When the coronary artery communicates with the right cardiac system through the fistula, the aortic blood is introduced into the right heart and mixed with the venous blood. The naming of CAVF is appropriate. However, when the blood is drained into the left cardiac system, because the aortic blood flows into the systemic circulation/cardiac cavity, the name of CAVF is inappropriate. In 1978, Perloff JK believed that it was best to use the name of congenital CAF. In 1982, Papaioannou A adopted the nomenclature of coronary systemic fistula.

3. History of CAF

In 1851, Austrian anatomist Josef H first reported this coronary artery abnormality. In 1865, Krause W described the congenital malformation of CAF in detail (Figure 1-7), and then Haller JA and Little JA also described the clinical triad signs of CAF, including cardiac murmur, left-right atrial or ventricular shunt, and large tortuous coronary arteries.

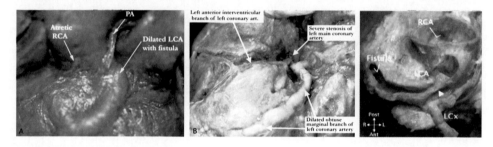

Figure 1-7 Autopsy changes of CAF. A: LCA-RV fistula with dilated LCA; B: LCA-LV fistula with coronary atherosclerotic disease (CAD); C: LCA-RV fistula.

In 1912, Trevor RS reported the first patient with CAF from RCA to RV by autopsy. The first surgery was performed in 1947 by Bjork G and Crafoord C, in which they closed CAF terminating in PA on a 15-year-old patient with a pre-operative diagnosis of PDA. Almost 20 years later, in 1963, the first successful coronary artery bypass grafting (CABG) was performed by Cooley DA and Hallman GL in order to treat fistula between LCA and RV.

The first surgical treatment of CAF was completed with the assistance of cardiopulmonary bypass (CPB) by Swan H in 1959. In 1983, Reidy JF was the first to report TCC of CAF, and it was minimally invasive with fast recovery and other advantages compared with surgical thoracotomy. If TCC is contraindicated, surgical closure or ligation of the fistula is implemented.

In the past 40 years, many clinicians at home and abroad have conducted comparative studies on these 2 methods (Figure 1-8).

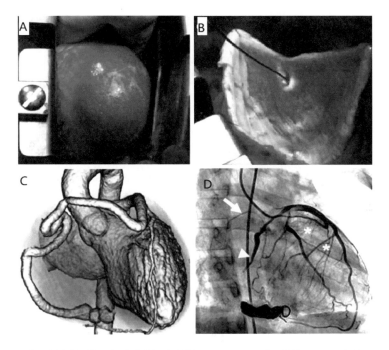

Figure 1-8   A & B: Surgical field of RCA aneurysm; C: CTA showed the anterior course of the separate RCA coming off LAD; D: One year after coil embolization, selective ICA clearly distinguished the contrast effect of LAD and LCX, the sinus node branch from LCX (white arrow), and RV branches from RCA (asterisks). The proximal end of the coil-embolized CAF formed a thrombus (arrowhead).

4. Etiology and classification

Congenital CAF is mainly caused by the continuous opening of the myocardial trabecular sinus space. During early fetal development, sinusoids nourish the primitive myocardium, connected to the tubular heart. Later in adulthood, sinusoids normally become obliterated into the Thebesian vessels and capillaries. Persistent sinusoids may contribute to fistulous communication between the coronary arteries and cardiac chambers (CCF). On the other hand, the remnant connection between coronary arteries and other mediastinal vessels (i.e. bronchial, pericardial, or mediastinal arteries) or the superior vena cava (SVC) may cause congenital CAVF.

Acquired CAF develops from iatrogenic or traumatic events, with a predominance of the former, including the followings: heart transplant and biopsy, mitral valve replacement, percutaneous coronary intervention (PCI), septal myectomy, closed-chest ablation, chest irradiation, CABG, permanent pacemaker placement, several diseases [i. e. infective endocarditis (IE), coronary vasculitis, and AMI], and transbronchial lung biopsy. However, acquired CAF due to traumatic injury can occur in both thorax penetrating and non-penetrating accidents. In these cases, the most common origin is RCA, and the most common termination is the right chambers of the heart. Although acquired CAF is rare, the incidence is increasing with the growth of cardiovascular surgery and other treatment procedures.

CAF is a kind of abnormal end of coronary artery, also known as an anomaly of coronary termination. The main or branches of the left and right coronary arteries directly enter the cardiac cavity, PA, CS, pulmonary veins, SVC, bronchial vessels, etc. (Figures 1-9, 1-10, 1-11, and 1-12).

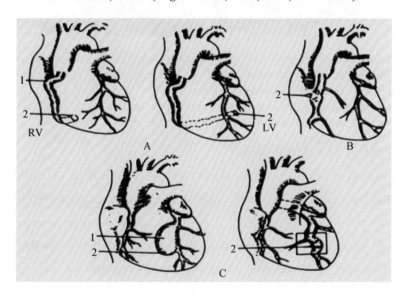

Figure 1-9   Schematic diagram of CAF. A: Coronary artery-RV fistula and coronary artery-LV fistula; B: Multiple fistulas of RCA; C: LAD-RV fistula. 1: Abnormal pathological coronary artery (fistula duct); 2: Fistula outlet.

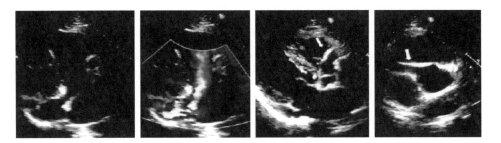

Figure 1-10   Echo changes of congenital RCA-CS fistula.

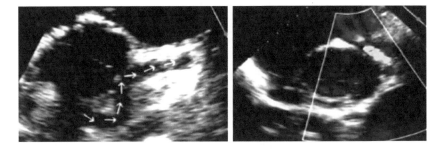

Figure 1-11   Echo changes of acquired LCA-RV fistula after surgery for tetralogy of Fallot (TOF).

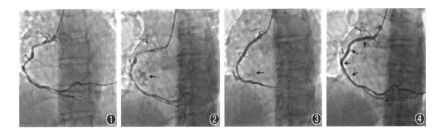

Figure 1-12   ① ICA showed 75% diffuse stenosis of RCA; ② RCA-RV fistula was caused by perforation of guidewire; ③ Fistula shunt decreased after stent implantation; ④ Spontaneous complete closure 7 months after stent implantation.

CAA is best described in the dog, hamster, and cow though reports also exist in the horse and pig. The most well-known anomaly in veterinary medicine is anomalous coronary artery origin with a pre-pulmonary course in dogs, which limits the treatment of pulmonary valve stenosis.

Similar to humans, fistulas in mammals, especially cattle, usually occur between the coronary arteries and ventricles of the heart. In addition to cattle, canine CAF may also be congenital or secondary to trauma, IE, mycotic infection, or atherosclerosis.

5. Morphology of CAF

While the exact percentage of morphological origins and terminations of CAF differ, the consensus is that fistulas are typically found on the right side of the heart. Studies showed that the origin of 52% of CAF is RCA, 30% at LAD, and 18% at LCX. Regardless of origin, nearly 90% of fistulas drain to the right chambers of the heart, most frequently to RV in about 40%, followed by RA, CS, and pulmonary trunk. Fistulas that originate proximally and drain into RA are much more dilated but less tortuous. The most anatomically complex CAF are those that originate from RCA and drain into CS with extremely large size and tortuous.

In 1974, a study by Ogden JA was the first to categorize CAF based on their drainage site in the atriums, classifying them into 3 types (Figure 1-13).

Type 1 can either terminate into RA or LA and these fistulas are physiologically similar to each other but different from those terminating in the high pressure ventricles. The thick walls of the ventricles allow for the closure of the fistula during ventricular systole, whereas the thinner walls of the atriums do not affect the fistula opening. Type 1 classically has short, dilated arterial branches that extend from RCA and terminate in either the right appendage or RA vestibule. RA-terminating (Type 1) CAF usually only involves RCA, whereas those terminating in LA mainly involve LCA.

Type 2 is the most frequently encountered and is more variable than Type 1, since both LCA and RCA can feed the fistula. From its point of origin, the fistula usually travels posteriorly between the atriums and drains at a point anterior to SVC. If it does not terminate at SVC, CAF will travel around SVC and terminate into the posterior surface of the atrium.

Type 3 includes CAF that terminates in the posterior surface of RA or LA, usually along the atrioventricular groove. As with Type 2, Type 3 can involve either RCA or LCA. However, the termination of the fistula

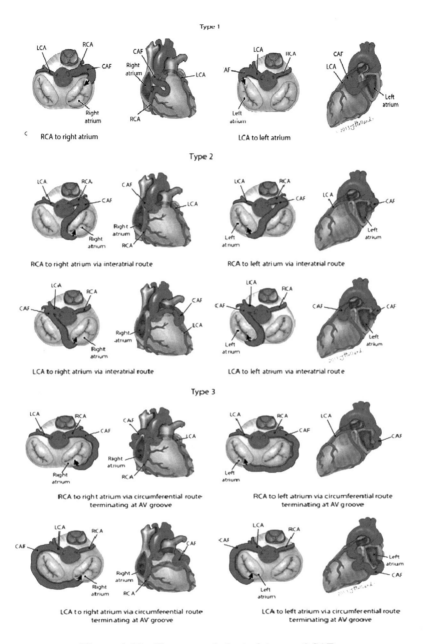

Figure 1-13　Three morphological types of CAF.

determines the blood flow during diastole and systole. If the CAF terminates in RV, it will pass through the myocardium and be closed upon systolic contraction and will cause increased hemodynamic stress on the heart. The far less hemodynamic difference is seen in fistulas terminating in LV. However, if the origin of the fistula is LCA and it terminates in LA, the overall pressure in LA will increase compared to those terminating in RA. While hemodynamic changes can cause serious complications, several studies hypothesize that collateral circulation from the uninvolved coronary artery compensates for blood loss to the chambers and prevents AMI.

6. Anatomy of CAF

CAF may originate from either RCA or LCA, and it is rare to have both coronary arteries involved. The majority of the fistula arise from a coronary artery with an otherwise normal anatomic course. Proximal to the fistula, the coronary is often dilated and elongated in proportion to the shunt size across the fistulous communication. Distal to the fistula, the vessel usually returns to normal size (Figure 1-14).

Lowe JE reviewed 286 patients and found the most common origin was RCA, followed by LCA system. The right side of the heart was the most common drainage site in the following descending drainage site in the order: RV (39%), RA (33%, including CS and SVC), and PA (20%). LA or LV was the termination site in the remaining 8%.

Qureshi SA found that the fistula between the coronary artery and RV accounted for 41%, RA 26%, PA 17%, LV 3%, and SVC 1%. Iadanza A found that more than 90% of CAF form a connection with the venous system, resulting in the hemodynamic effect of left-right shunt. CAF can originate from the trunk and branches of any coronary artery, but it is more common in RCA and LAD, and other branches such as LCX are rare. Single CAF accounts for 74%–90%, and double CAF accounts for 10%–26%. RCA fistula is common, accounting for 50%–60%, LCA fistula is 30%–40%, and bilateral CAF is 10% (Figures 1-15, 1-16). The incidence of simple CAF is 55%–88%, and 20%–45% are accompanied by other various congenital heart diseases (CHD).

A review of the literature shows that there is no uniform consensus regarding the most common site of origin. However, LM is reported to be the

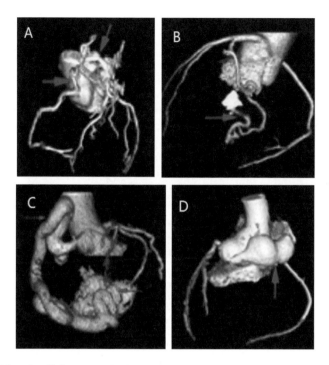

Figure 1-14　A: Volume rendering images showed tortuous and dilated fistula vessels communicating with RCA/LAD and PA, the left red arrow showed the fistula vessel from RCA, and the right red arrow showed the fistula vessel from LAD; B: The red arrow showed the fistula originating from LCX and draining into LV; C: Tortuous and dilated RCA communicating with RA, the left red arrow indicated the tortuous and dilated RCA, and the right red arrow indicated the drainage site of RA; D: Volume rendering image showed AN in LAD (red arrow).

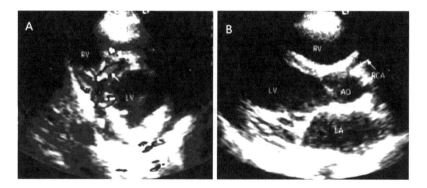

Figure1-15　Echo findings of RCA-RV fistula. A: Turbulence signals of multiple fistula openings in the RV (white arrow); B: The dilated RCA (white arrow).

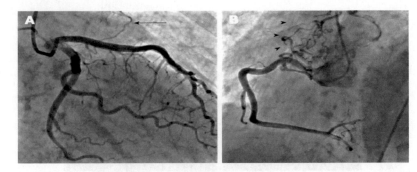

Figure 1-16　ICA findings of bilateral fistulas.　A:　LAD-PA fistula with single origin, multiple pathway and single termination (arrow); B: RCA-PA fistula with multiple origin, pathway and termination (arrowheads).

most common origin in several studies, whereas the most common site of drainage is PA.　Most CAPF identified on CTA have a favorable prognosis. Observation with optimal medical treatment (OMT) is usually an appropriate strategy.　Fistula size is a possible determinant for surgical treatment.

7. Histology and pathology of CAF

In order to study the histology of CAF, Neufeld HN removed a segment of the parent coronary artery involved in a fistula that terminated in RV. Microscopic analysis showed that most of the vessels had prominent muscle bundles and contained a duplicated internal elastic lamina dispersed between them.　Additionally,　the　tunica　intima　layer　had　nonspecific　fibrous thickening.

8. Pathophysiological consequences

As a very rare cardiac anomaly, CAF is also the most hemodynamically significant lesion affecting the cardiovascular system.　Approximately half of CAF patients are asymptomatic,　and　some　congenital fistulas may be spontaneously closed during childhood.　The symptoms of chest pain and exertional dyspnea are often due to the progressive enlargement of CAF and increasing volume of left-right shunt.　There is a relationship between the anomalous origin of LCA from PA and anterolateral AMI in newborns. However, because the coronary vessels primarily supply metabolic support to the dependent myocardium, physiological alterations in this function should be the main consideration. Although the clinical presentation of CAF varies widely, it depends on the size of the fistula, the age of the patient, and the presence of myocardial ischemia.

CHF was also very common and mainly attributed to volume overload secondary to multiple CAF and large shunt. They also suggested that although pulmonary hypertension has been reported to be the cause of dyspnea in some patients and exertional angina without angiographic evidence of CAD has been attributed to a coronary steal phenomenon. This phenomenon suggests a decrease in myocardial perfusion on exertion due to the inability of the coronary flow reserve (Figure 1-17).

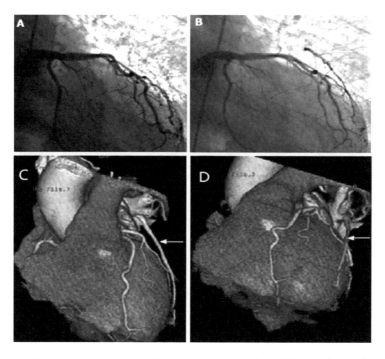

Figure 1-17   A 67-year-old man admitted to the hospital with exertional chest pain for 6 weeks. A: Showed coronaries without significant atherosclerotic lesion; B, C & D: Showed fistula between LAD and superior pulmonary vein.

The pathophysiological characteristics and clinical manifestations are closely related to the size of CAF.

(1) Giant CAF have large involved vessels, often accompanied by

tortuous vessels and/or tumor-like dilation (AN).

a. Coronary blood volume increases with left-right shunt or coronary artery reflux to LV. In severe cases, the shunt flow can reach more than 20% of cardiac output. Continuous murmurs or diastolic murmurs (coronary artery-LV fistula) can be heard on precordial auscultation, leading to cardiac dilatation, CHF, and other clinical manifestations.

b. Because the involved vessel of CAF is large, the blood flow is fast, and the resistance is low, it often causes the blood flow of the normal coronary artery to decrease, and there is a coronary steal phenomenon, which is prone to clinical symptoms related to myocardial ischemia, such as angina, arrhythmia, and AMI.

c. Due to the increased blood flow at the proximal abnormal coronary artery, shearing force-induced vascular intimal damage and coronary atherosclerosis can occur. In addition, the involved vessels are tortuous and dilated, which are easy to cause thrombosis.

(2) Small CAF are often found by ICA due to chest pain and suspected CAD. Because the involved vessel is small, the shunt flow is slow, and the pathophysiological change is slight, there are no obvious clinical symptoms and signs.

(3) The pathophysiological characteristics and clinical manifestations of patients with intermediate CAF are between the above two.

9. Presentation and symptoms

Typically CAF is often asymptomatic during childhood. Based on several studies, symptoms are present in 19%–63% of patients, with the majority occurring after 18 or 20 years of age. The most common symptom reported is dyspnea on exertion. Murmurs are also commonly reported with CAF; many otherwise asymptomatic fistulas are often found after angiographic investigation of continuous murmurs heard at the left sternal border. Studies report that the majority of adult patients with CAF usually present with a murmur, whereas only 9% of children have continuous murmurs. When fistulas terminate in the left-sided chamber, the aortic run-off mimics aortic insufficiency and its murmur.

While paroxysmal nocturnal dyspnea and murmurs are the most prevalent among reported presentations, the followings are also reported: fatigue, atrial arrhythmia, pulmonary hypertension (PH), CHF, presence of AN, rupture or thrombosis of the fistula, pneumonia, palpitation, upper respiratory infection, hemoptysis, edema, IE, and angina. Angina experienced in CAF patients is usually seen when the fistula is combined with other cardiac anomalies, such as CAD, HOCM, and aortic stenosis.

Said SAM and his colleagues published a very meaningful paper. The authors retrospectively analyzed the clinical data of 304 cases of CAF in adults (47% male) worldwide. The average age is 51.4 (18–86) years old, and 20% are over 65 years old. Clinical manifestations: shortness of breath (31%), chest tightness or palpitation (23%), and angina (21%). Typical biphasic murmurs can be heard in 82% of patients. Chest X-ray can detect only 4%, while CT, Echo and ICA can detect 16%, 68% and 97% of the abnormalities, respectively. Among the patients with single fistulas, 69% came from LCA and 31% from RCA. 80% belonged to single fistulas, 18% had double fistulas, and 2% had multiple fistulas. Aneurysmal dilatation occurred in 14% of patients, and spontaneous rupture, pulmonary embolism and pericardial tamponade occurred in 2% of patients (Figure 1-18).

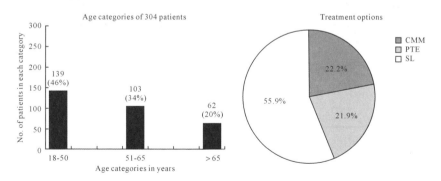

Figure 1-18   Age distribution and treatment strategy of 304 patients with CAF. CMM: Conservative medical management; PTE: Percutaneous therapeutic embolization; SL: Surgical ligation.

10. Complications

Though the majority of CAF are etiologically congenital, complications typically do not present until the age of 18 or 20. These complications display a wide range in severity, from being asymptomatic in 75% – 90% of cases to presenting with myocardial ischemia and aortic insufficiency. When present, symptoms are usually secondary to CHF, which, in turn, results from left-right shunt. Arrhythmia can also occur due to excessive cardiac chamber load, as well as CHF in older patients. IE have been reported in incidences varying from 0% to 12% (Figure 1-19), and 20% of patients with CAF, and additional cardiac anomalies have also been reported. These anomalies include TOF, aortic atresia, pulmonary atresia, ASD, VSD, and PDA. In rare cases, the initial manifestation was myocardial ischemia, pericardial effusion, or sudden death. Lozano I reported a patient whose cardiac catheterization revealed multiple small fistulas from LAD to LV, with normal systolic function. And this patient had an ICD implanted due to a documented ventricular fibrillation (VF) episode.

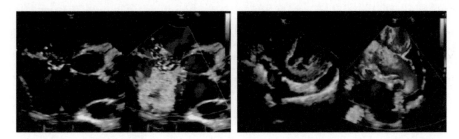

Figure 1-19   Echo changes of LCA-RV fistula with IE.

11. Diagnostics

Due to the asymptomatic nature of CAF, many incidental findings are found during routine examinations. Some patients can accompany with LV and RV overload or hypertrophy on ECG examination. CAF draining into CS and RA are prone to atrial fibrillation, and a few patients have myocardial ischemic changes such as ST segment depression, and T wave inversion. The gold standard for identifying CAF remains ICA; however, non-invasive two-

and three-dimensional imaging techniques are becoming more common. The benefit of ICA is that it can determine which coronary artery is involved in the fistula. Based on this, it can help to identify the communicating chamber or vessel and the locations of CAF with respect to the proximal/distal portions of the vessel. Although ICA acts as the standard for CAF diagnosis, new methods including multidetector CT (MDCT) or multislice CT (MSCT), MR, TEE, TTE, and color Doppler flow imaging (CDFI) have also been beneficial (Figures 1-20, 1-21).

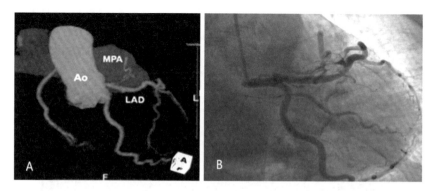

Figure 1-20   CT and angiographic examination of LAD-PA fistula.

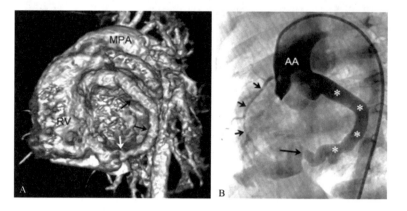

Figure 1-21   CCF between LCX and RV in a 1-month-old boy. A: CT image showed the diffusely dilated LCX (arrows) anomalously connecting to RV; B: Aortographic image showed the dilated LCX (asterisks) draining into RV (long arrow). A normal RCA (short arrows) was noted. AA: Ascending aorta; MPA: Main pulmonary artery.

TEE provides a good view of the structures at the base of the heart, and with this approach, the anatomy of the fistula (origin and its termination) can often be visualized. Additionally, high-resolution transducers can often display the cardiac vessels with greater spatial resolution than other imaging methods, allowing evaluation of blood flow in the fistula. However, TEE is lack of detection of the aberrant fistulas on the right side of the heart.

Utilizing the combination of pulsed and two-dimensional CDFI in suspected or confirmed cases of CAF, coronary artery dilation, termination chamber, and turbulent flow can be observed. The non-invasive CDFI is a tremendous benefit, allowing it to be used to monitor the status of the fistula. Additionally, CDFI is often utilized to determine the severity of blood shunt (Figure 1-22). Along with a high frequency transducer, transthoracic CDFI allows for the visualization of multiple microfistulas from the coronary artery to LV.

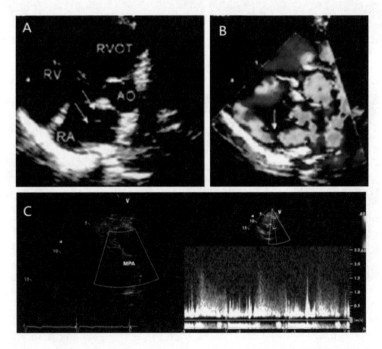

Figure 1-22　TEE and CDFI of RCA-RA fistula (A & B) and LAD-PA fistula (C).

If surgery for CAF proves necessary, TEE can be used to determine the precise drainage site. TEE is an invaluable tool, as the precise termination points are often not detectable through pre-operative ICA.

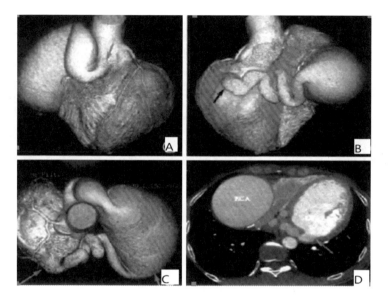

Figure 1-23 CT findings of RCA-LV fistula and AN.

Other imaging techniques including CT and MR scan have been used for both diagnostics and follow-up (Figure 1-23). In the last decade, MDCT or MSCT and ICA have gained clinical significance in CAF diagnostics due to their ability to provide detailed images with minimally invasive techniques. MDCT can provide superior visualization of CAF, possible AN, and adjacent anatomical structures. In addition to MDCT, MR can determine what coronary vessels are involved in CAF, such as the location, course, blood flow, and function of the fistula.

(1) Pediatric CAF

As in the general population, most pediatric patients were asymptomatic, and the majority of fistulas were congenital (Figure 1-24). Only several patients had acquired fistulas as a consequence of TOF repair and others. In addition to TOF, other cardiac anomalies in the pediatric patient cohort were PDA and ASD. While post-operative angiographic studies deemed the surgical repair successful, Mavroudis C set out to determine whether coil embolization should be performed as an alternative therapy. Based on their research, the criterion of coil occlusion was established:

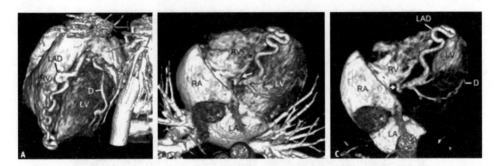

Figure 1-24   CCF between LAD and RV in a 5-year-old boy. A: CT image showed the diffusely dilated LAD and D branch; B & C: CT images with a full slab (B) and with a thinner slab (C) demonstrated the single drainage site (arrows) of the fistula into the inferomedial basal portion of RV.

    a. the presence of only one CAF;

    b. a narrow drainage site upon termination;

    c. the absence of large branch vessels;

    d. relatively safe access to the involved coronary artery of the fistula.

Kothandam S reported 3 CHF cases(an 8-year-old girl weighing 20 kg, a 3-year-old boy weighing 10 kg, and a 9-month-old infant weighing 5 kg) with large CAF draining to the left heart structures (Figures 1-25, 1-26).

(2) Prenatal CAF

CAF accounts for 50% of pediatric coronary vascular aberrations, and it is believed to originate from the Thebesian vessels. During prenatal life, the coronary arteries communicate with the ventricles via intratrabecular spaces. As the fetus develops, these intratrabecular spaces become sinusoids that communicate between the coronary arteries, veins and heart chambers. Fistulas are thought to develop if these intratrabecular spaces are not close to sinusoids.

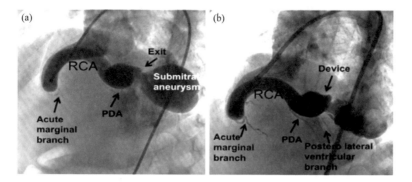

Figure 1-25 A large end-artery fistula from the distal RCA exits into LV where it forms a localized sub-mitral aneurysm. (a) Following the closure of the narrow distal exit with ventricular septal occluder; (b) The coronary branches fill well.

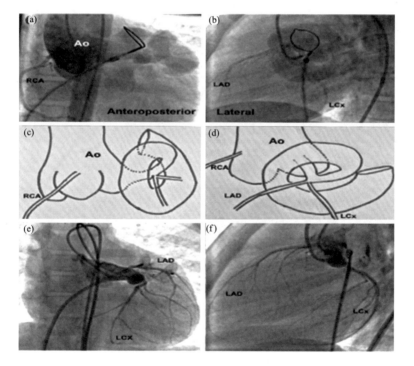

Figure 1-26 ICA in anteroposterior (a) and lateral (b) views showed large fistula from LCA to the left atrial appendage (LAA). Cartoon representation (c & d) showed a narrower first part that turns superiorly to the second broader part and finally turns inferiorly to the third larger part before draining into LA. After closure (e & f) with 2 plugs, there is no residual flow.

Imaging techniques can now be used to diagnose CAF prenatally, enabling swift treatment if the left-right shunt poses a significant hemodynamic problem to the heart. While these imaging techniques can be beneficial, fetal cardiac vessels are difficult to discern based on the size and movement of the heart.

Gurleen K carried out a retrospective review of 5 babies diagnosed prenatally with CAF (Figure 1-27). Lai QR reported 7 cases of fetal CAF (Figures 1-28, 1-29). Echo features and measurements were noted during pregnancy and after births, and treatments and outcomes were also noted.

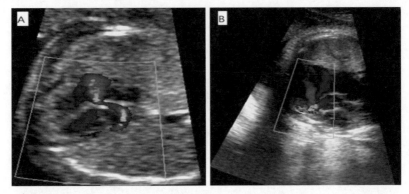

Figure 1-27　A: CAF from LCA to LA; B: CAF from RCA to RA.

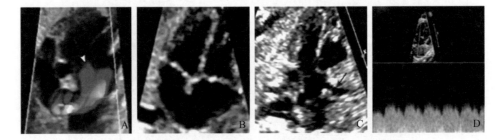

Figure 1-28　Echo findings of RCA-RA fistula. The woman was 23-year-old and 32 weeks pregnant. A: Abnormal blood flow bundle from aortic root to RA (arrowhead); B: There was no change in the size of fetal cardiac cavities; C: Trace the flow bundle, and the dilated RCA (black arrow) at the root of the aorta, with an opening of 3.3 mm and the widest part of 4.6 mm, which is tortuous; D: The drainage site is the anterior edge of right atrial septum, and the flow velocity is 3.71 m/s. The spectrum characteristics are similar to the blood flow spectrum of children's PDA, which is two-phase continuous blood flow.

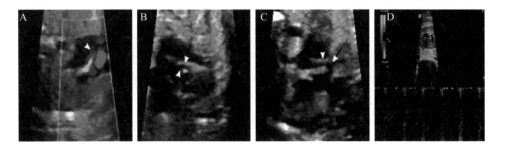

Figure 1-29 Echo findings of LCA-RA fistula. The woman was 34-year-old and 23
weeks pregnant. A: Abnormal blood flow bundle (arrow) is seen in RA, and the root
of the autonomic artery enters RA; B: Tracking the flow bundle, the beginning of the
dilated LCA (arrow) can be seen; C: Dilated LCA (arrow); D: The Doppler spectrum
of abnormal blood flow is similar to that of PDA in children, which is continuous
biphasic blood flow mainly in diastole.

Although CAF can be diagnosed accurately during fetal life, some babies may
develop CHF shortly after birth and need early treatment. Patients with
conservative treatment should continue to be followed-up, because TCC or
surgical intervention may be required in the future.

Several studies on prenatal diagnosis revealed that CAF and other
suspected cardiac anomalies were found using CDFI, such as ASD. CDFI
often confirms the existence of CAF, and pulsed Doppler can determine
blood flow through the fistula. Prenatally diagnosed CAF can be monitored
throughout pregnancy using Echo. After birth, ICA can confirm the
diagnosis.

As techniques and guidelines become more and more advanced and
feasible, early intervention and higher survival rate for prenatally diagnosed
cases may occur. Prenatal imaging allows for the proper perinatal follow-up
and diligent monitoring of cardiac complications.

(3) Acquired CAF

Chronic total occlusion (CTO) is the most challenging case in PCI. In
recent years, with the accumulation of operator experiences and the
improvement of instruments, the incidence of complications in patients with
CTO during hospitalization has decreased significantly. At Mayo Clinic, the

peri-operative mortality and incidence of AMI decreased significantly. Emergent CABG decreased from 15% in 1979 to 3% in 2005. Twenty-five years of observation showed that serious adverse cardiac events tended to decrease, but the incidence of pericardial tamponade caused by CAP remained at 1% .

CAP is reported to be directly proportional to the complexity of coronary artery disease. Risk factors can be categorized as followings:

a. Non-modifiable risk factors

—Old age;

—Female gender;

—History of previous CABG;

—Use of clopidogrel.

b. Modifiable risk factors

—Presence of hypertension;

—Presence of peripheral artery disease;

—Presence of CHF;

—Lower body mass index (BMI);

—Lower creatinine clearance.

c. Risk factors associated with coronary anatomy and catheterization

—Complex coronary lesions (ACC/AHA Type B2, C);

—CTO, heavily calcified lesions, angulated, tortuous lesions, and narrow coronary arteries;

—Aggressive use of oversized balloons and stents;

—Use of atheroablative devices and hydrophilic guidewires.

Mikhail P demonstrated that CAP occurs in approximately 1 in 250 "all-comer" PCI procedures, and the overall incidence is fairly steady. Still catastrophic perforations (Ellis Ⅲ) have been more common in recent years; perforation mortality is fairly low but not insignificant (7.5%) and has declined over time; female sex, kidney disease, previous CABG, hypertension, and LAD target vessel are important clinical risk factors for CAP. Finally, most coronary perforations are successfully managed with balloon tamponade or covered stents without the requirement for surgical intervention (Figure 1-30).

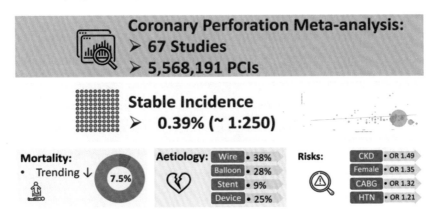

Figure 1-30   The detailed systematic review of the largest comprehensive overview of patients with PCI-related CAP.

Twenty-nine studies met pre-specified inclusion criteria reporting the etiology of CAP (n = 1,242). Coronary guidewires were the most frequent cause of CAP during PCI (37.3%) of reported perforations. Balloon dilatation pre- and post-stent deployment accounted for 27.5% , with stent deployment accounting for 24.4% and other devices causing 9.1% of CAP (Figure 1-31A).

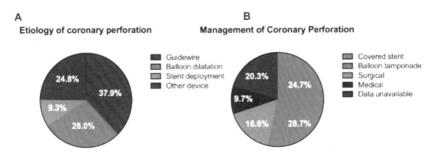

Figure 1-31   Etiology and management of CAP.

Surgical management was required in 16.6% of patients with CAP. Approximately half of CAP could be managed percutaneously with balloon or covered stent. Conservative management was successfully used as the only treatment in 9.7% of CAP without percutaneous or surgical intervention. The final treatment modality for CAP was indeterminate in 20.3% of analyzed patients preventing further analysis in this subgroup (Figure 1-31B). Of the cases where the final treatment modality was available, CAP was managed with covered stents for 31%, balloon tamponade in 36%, surgically in 21%, and medically in 12% of cases.

Incidence is reported to be low and can vary between 0.1% and 3% based on the several case series with the highest risk of CAP occurring while dealing with CTO. Mortality can be as high as 21.2%, depending on the severity of CAP. Distal CAP can be sealed with combined coil and fat, absorbable suture, etc.

O'Sullivan D described the case of an 86-year-old man with an extensive cardiac history, including previous CABG, who experienced a delayed extracardiac hematoma, 350 ml in volume, after retrograde CTO-PCI. The patient was successfully treated with the resultant liquefaction of the hematoma (Figure 1-32).

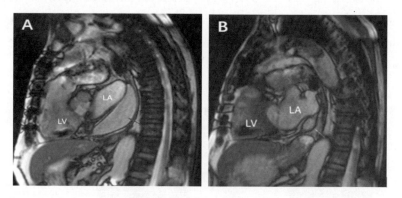

Figure 1-32 A: CMR demonstrated an extracardiac hematoma (red arrow) compressing LA; B: 3 months (blue arrows) after CAP.

Chen D reported the case of CAP complicating Bioresorbable Vascular Scaffold (BVS) implantation and the associated technical challenges with managing this life-threatening complication (Figure 1-33).

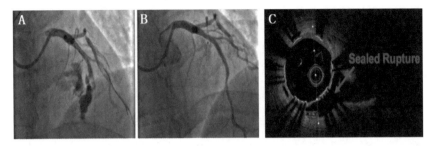

Figure 1-33 A: Large Ellis type Ⅲ CAP at the distal edge of the BVS with no flow to distal LAD beyond the rupture. Prolonged balloon inflation immediately proximal to the site of perforation combined with fluid and vasopressor support achieved hemodynamic stability; B: A 3.0 mm × 21 mm BeGraft covered stent deployed across the perforation distal to the diagonal side-branch at 14 atm, with approximately 10 mm of overlap between the Absorb BVS and the covered stent; C: OCT demonstrated very short segment of malapposition of BeGraft in Absorb BVS at proximal overlap margin.

Sugitani M presented the case of a 75-year-old man who experienced rebleeding after surgical treatment of type Ⅲ CAP, resulting in intertwined complications, including communicating coronary and ventricular pseudoaneurysms. The PCI of sealing the rebleeding site with covered stent implantation managed this rare pseudoaneurysm successfully (Figure 1-34).

Yanagisawa S reported the case of an 82-year-old man who was indicated for cardiac resynchronization therapy (CRT) and underwent left bundle branch area pacing. The patient had no chest symptoms during or after implantation. Post-operative Echo demonstrated a new abnormal tunnel inside the IVS and shunt flow from the IVS toward the RV. ICA confirmed a septal CAF, which might have been formed by failed deep screw attempts. Since the shunt volume assessed by the Qp/Qs was small, the patient was treated conservatively (Figure 1-35).

Wang XW Reported a case of LAA-coronary artery fistula caused by LAA occlusion (Figure 1-36).

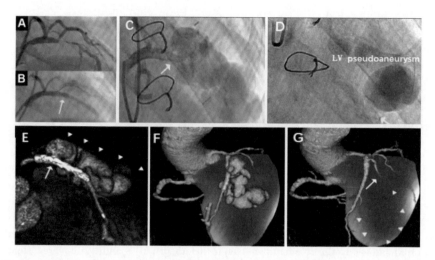

Figure 1-34   A: ICA revealed a bifurcation lesion in the mid-LAD; B: An Ellis type Ⅲ CAP occurred (yellow arrow); C & D: ICA showed the communicating pseudoaneurysms with the rebleeding site and the fistula draining into LV (arrows); E: CT showed the communicating pseudoaneurysms (arrowheads) connected with LAD (yellow arrows); F & G: An anterior perfusion defect (yellow arrowheads), which is corresponding to the pseudoaneurysm-induced diagonal occlusion (white arrow) on fused SPECT/CT images.

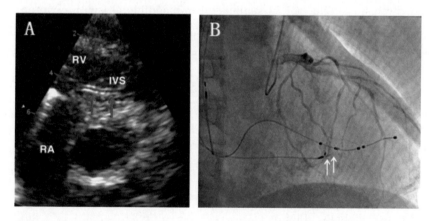

Figure 1-35   Post-operative Echo and ICA. A: Echo after implantation revealed an abnormal tunnel with a diameter of 1.2 mm inside IVS (red arrow); B: ICA showed a large septal branch extending into the lower IVS and septal artery fistula to the RV septum around the RV lead (white arrow).

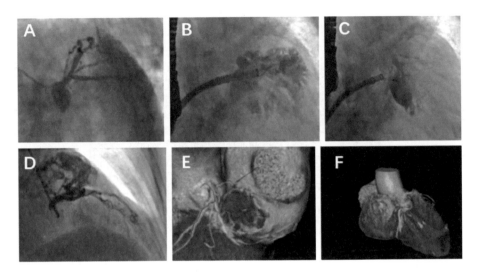

Figure 1-36   A: ICA showed normal LCX without fistula; B & C: LAA closure; D: Angiogram showed LCX-LAA fistula; E & F: CTA showed 2 small branches of the proximal part of LCX to the anterior wall of LAA, and occluder shadow can be seen in good shape.

12. Treatment

A single fistula is more common, accounting for up to 90% of all CAF, and 75% of incidentally found CAF are clinically silent. Since CAF mostly remains asymptomatic, the treatment of CAF is essentially medical and conservative management with continued follow-up (Figure 1-37). While rare, some authors reported several cases of spontaneous closure of CAF without surgical or catheter repair. Among these, most spontaneous closures occur in children diagnosed with CAF before 2 years of age, and these fistulas almost always drain into RV.

Iwaki T reported a case of spontaneous closure of CAF with familial hypercholesterolemia (Figure 1-38).

(1) Surgery techniques

Surgical correction of CAF in asymptomatic patients is controversial. When fistulas are detected in young patients, several studies believe it best to repair the fistula prior to developing more serious complications. The main indication for closure of the fistula is the existence of a significant left-right

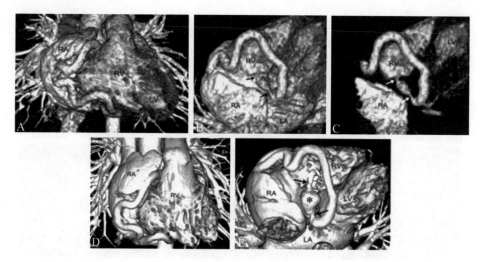

Figure 1-37 CCF between RCA and RV. A: CT image showed the diffusely dilated RCA in a 5-month-old boy; B & C: CT images with a full slab (B) and with a thinner slab (C) demonsted the single drainage site of the fistula into the inferomedial basal portion of RV. Two narrowings (arrows) are noted at the drainage site. D & E: Follow-up frontal (D) and inferior (E) volume-rendered CT images (8 years later) showed increased dilatation of RCA and the development of aneurysmal change (asterisk) at the drainage site. The 2 narrowings (arrows) showed interval increase in diameter due to left-right shunt through the fistula.

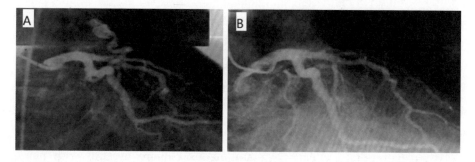

Figure 1-38 ICA of spontaneous closure of LAD-PA fistula. A: The angiographic image at the age of 43 showed fistula; B: At the age of 51, the fistula disappeared.

shunt that causes ventricular overload (Figure 1-39). This shunt is commonly known as the coronary steal phenomenon, in which the blood movement from a high-pressure fistula into a low-pressure chamber causes hemodynamic stress on the heart. If severe, coronary steal phenomenon can cause extreme

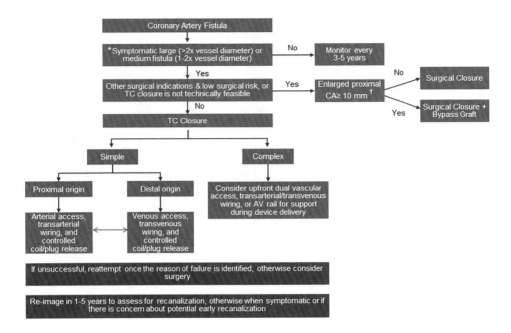

Figure 1-39   Algorithm of CAF evaluation and management.

∗ Symptomatic fistulas are CAF that potentially leads to myocardial ischemia, AN and rupture, IE, unexplained cardiac chamber enlargement/dysfunction, or arrhythmia.

†An enlarged proximal coronary artery with diameter $\geqslant 10$ mm has a tendency to thrombus after fistula closure, resulting in AMI. A simple fistula has a single-vessel origin, simply defined pathways, and a clearly defined termination. A complex fistula is a large fistula with multiple origins and plexiform formation. AV: arteriovenous; TC: transcatheter.

cardiac damage including hypertrophy, as well as ischemia due to re-routing of the coronary vessels.

Treatment options remain controversial, if large shunt is present but do not cause pathological problems or symptoms. If large shunt and AN are detected in the pediatric patients, they are usually corrected in order to avoid late complications (Figure 1-40). In fact, retrospective reviews concluded that complications involved in surgical correction outweighed the risk of CAF itself. In an extremely mild shunt, however, Cheung DL suggested that regular screening to monitor pathological changes should be utilized prior to

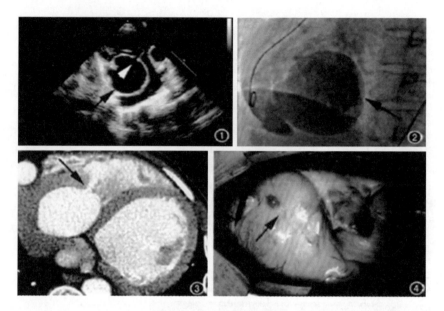

Figure 1-40　Imaging examination and surgical field of RCA-RV fistula. ① Echo findings; ② Angiographic findings; ③ CT showed AN; ④ Surgical field.

elective surgical correction. Li H reported a rare case of giant LCX with fistula formation treated with successful surgery (Figures 1-41, 1-42).

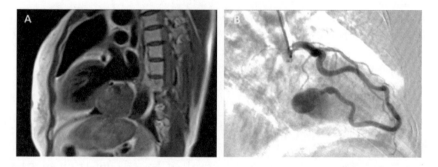

Figure 1-41　Pre-operative MR examination and ICA. A: MRI showed a mixed mass in the left atrioventricular groove area, accompanied by LA compression; B: ICA showed coronary atherosclerosis with a large LCX communicating with LA.

　　In CAF patients whose operative correction proves necessary, surgical ligation or TCC are possible treatment options. The type of operative correction for CAF depends on the location of the fistula, the involved coronary artery, and the termination of the connection. Direct ligation of the

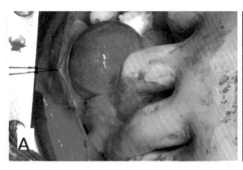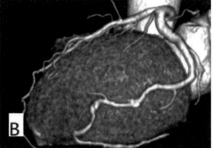

Figure 1-42   The giant AN during surgery. A: A giant round AN (4.2 cm × 5.5 cm × 6.4 cm) with an intact capsule and no adhesion to surrounding tissues was found on the surface of LV near the atrioventricular groove; B: CTA examination 3.5 years after the surgery showed CAD but no evidence of AN or LA fistula.

fistula at the drainage site is typically preferred because it eliminates the possibility of myocardial ischemia. However, if direct ligation of the coronary artery jeopardizes blood flow to the myocardium, grafting of the involved distal coronary artery is suggested.

Before these coronary bypass techniques were developed, surgical correction of CAF contained direct ligation or tangential arteriorrhaphy. Ligation was associated with high mortality, but arteriorrhaphy could be performed without CPB. For this procedure, multiple horizontal mattress sutures were placed between the coronary artery and the fistula to ensure that blood flows through the coronary artery remained unobstructed.

Lacona GM applied a new surgical technique in 7 adult patients: proximal and distal fistula closure, the opening of aneurysmal artery, and revascularization of branches rising from the fistula under CPB (Figures 1-43, 1-44).

Cubas WS presented the extremely rare case of LCX aneurysm with CAF to CS in a 20-year-old male patient, requiring surgical management due to the clinical presentation of this unusual condition (Figure 1-45).

Zhang SW reported a 22-year-old female with RCA-LV fistula underwent recanalization after surgery and then successfully performed interventional closure (Figure 1-46).

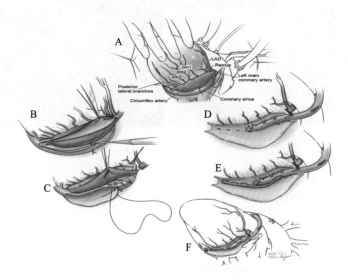

Figure 1-43 Surgical steps of the "Pettersson Repair". A: Initial view of LCX fistula; B: Dividing LCX and CS; C: Closing CS longitudinally; D: Ramus branch anastomosed to LAD and 3 OM revascularized with sequential vein anastomoses; E: 3 distal PL revascularized with sequential anastomoses using the free left internal thoracic artery graft, which is itself anastomosed to the vein graft; F: Final operative result.

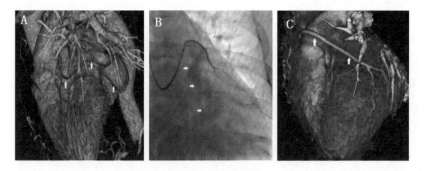

Figure 1-44 Pre-operative CTA (A) and ICA (B) indicated tortuous fistula between LCX and CS (arrows); Post-operative CTA (C) indicated the venous bypass graft feeding the coronary branches (arrows).

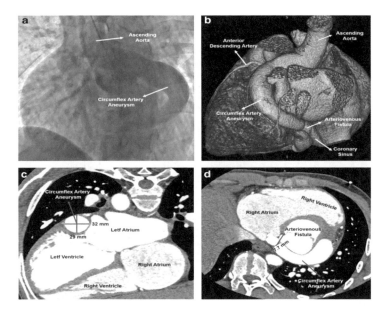

Figure 1-45 a: ICA with evidence of dilation of the LMCA and AN of LCX; b: CT showed aneurysmal LCX with fistulous connection to CS; c & d: CT showed measurements of AN and CAF respectively.

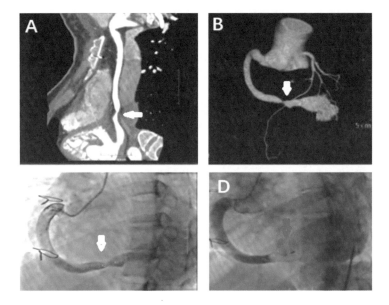

Figure 1-46 A: CT and ICA showed recanalization from RCA to LV after surgery (white arrow); D: ICA showed interventional plugging (red arrow).

(2) TCC techniques

Many studies suggest that TCC approaches are more beneficial than surgical approaches for eligible CAF cases (Figure 1-47). TCC techniques do not require median sternotomy or CPB, thus limiting potential iatrogenic complications.

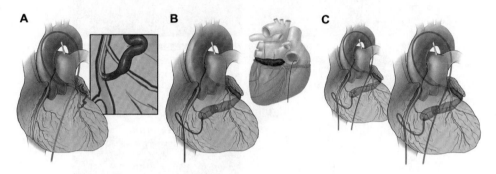

Figure 1-47 Three TCC techniques.
A: Transarterial approach. The coronary vessel is intubated, and the fistula is wired from its origin. The delivery catheter can then be delivered to the fistula over a wire for device deployment. The occlusion device is then deployed and released; B: Transvenous approach. The fistula termination site is intubated with the delivery catheter. The delivery catheter is advanced over a wire to the appropriate landing zone. The occlusion device is then deployed and released; C: Arteriovenous (AV) loop approach. In large and tortuous fistula, AV rail can be formed with the aid of a snare device to maximize support for catheter and device delivery.

TCC is also a less expensive procedure with lower morbidity, shorter recovery time, and better cosmetic results. On the other hand, the use of TCC approaches and coil occlusion techniques can also result in distal embolization or dissection of the fistula (Figures 1-48, 1-49 and 1-50).

Since 1983, several techniques and new products have been used. These products included covered stainless-steel coils, detachable balloons, Gianturco coils, platinum micro-coils, double umbrella devices, Amplatzer duct occluder, Gianturco Grifka vascular occlusion device, and so on. The type of occlusion device depends both on the surgeon's preference and the anatomical features of the fistula. Depending on the tortuosity, length, and dilation of the fistula, catheters with varying degrees of flexibility are

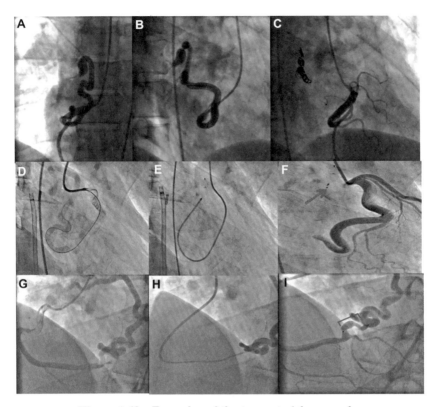

Figure 1-48   Examples of the transarterial approach.

A-C: A 53-year-old patient with a recent history of ACS. A: ICA demonstrated a proximal RCA-SVC fistula with a single origin and a tortuous pathway; B: Selective intubation of the fistula with a multipurpose (MP) guiding catheter was performed; C: After guidewire crossing and microcatheter positioning, two 4 mm/2 mm Tornado coils and three 14 mm × 6 mm Nester coils were released with excellent results. D-F: A 45-year-old woman with supraventricular tachycardia and a large distal fistula from LCX to SVC-RA junction. D: LCX was successfully wired using an 0.035-inch extra-stiff angled guidewire after failing to wire the fistula from the venous side; E: A 5-F, 125 cm MP diagnostic catheter was delivered deep into the fistula and an 8 mm Amplatzer vascular plug (AVP) Ⅳ was deployed; F: ICA 5 min after protamine administration to enhance clotting of AVP device (red arrow) illustrated absence of flow into the fistula. G-I: A 33-year-old man with a recent NSTEMI in the setting of a large distal RCA fistula to SVC. G: ICA with a 7-F Judkins guiding catheter demonstrated a large RCA with distal tortuous fistula emptying into SVC; H: The coaxial 90 cm Judkins guiding catheter and a 5-F, 125 cm MP catheter were successfully advanced to intubate the fistula over a 0.035-inch angled guidewire; I: An 8 mm AVP-Ⅳ device was successfully deployed in the proximal portion of the fistula away from the distal RCA branches.

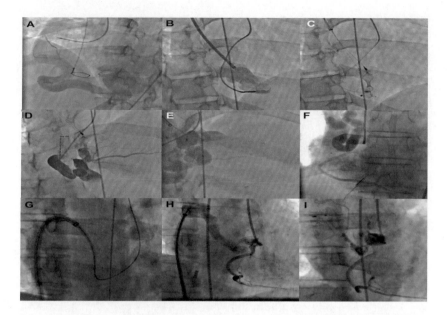

Figure 1-49 Examples of fistula closure with the aid of AV loop.

A-E: A 45-year-old patient with a large tortuous distal RCA communicating with the proximal CS. A: Transarterial wiring was successful, with a 0.014-inch Whisper guidewire after failure to advance a 0.035-inch angled guidewire through the tortuosity. A 5-F MP catheter and microcatheter were deeply intubated to provide support through the fistula termination. The wire was snared in the RA and exteriorized from the right internal jugular (RIJ) vein access with a snare. The microcatheter was advanced through RIJ sheath (kissing catheter and sheath), and the Whisper wire was switched for a supportive long-exchange 0.014-inch guidewire; B: The microcatheter was removed and a 7-F shuttle sheath was delivered through the venous access past the fistula termination; C: An 18 mm AVP-Ⅱ device was successfully deployed; D: ICA before release revealed that the device spanned the distal RCA branches. The device was retrieved and a smaller (14 mm) AVP-Ⅱ device was deployed; E: ICA revealed that the distal RCA branches were not at jeopardy with the 14 mm AVP-Ⅱ device. The device was successfully released afterward.

F-I: A 67-year-old woman with a history of IE and proximal RCA-SVC fistula. F: ICA demonstrated a tortuous fistula arising from the proximal RCA and emptying into SVC. The distal RCA was normal in size; G: Wiring the fistula through SVC was difficult. Therefore, transarterial wiring was performed with an exchange-length angled 0.035-inch guidewire that was exteriorized with the aid of a 4-F, 10 mm catheter. Over the created AV rail, an 8-F Cook Flexor sheath was delivered across the termination point of the fistula; H: ICA helped visualize the position of an 8/10 Amplatzer duct occluder (ADO-I); I: ICA after 5 min of partial reversal with Protamine showed no residual flow across the released ADO-I device (red star).

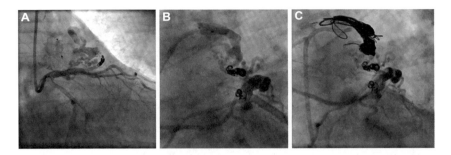

Figure 1-50　Example of transvenous approach.
A 65-year-old patient with a history of successful closure of simple RCA-PA fistula with AVP-Ⅱ device and unsuccessful closure of complex LAD-PA fistula with pushable coils. A: ICA revealed complex fistula with multiple origins and pathways arising from LAD and single termination into the main PA; B: The mouth of the fistula was successfully intubated through the venous access site with 7-F Amplatz guiding catheter; C: Three detachable coils were successfully released, abolishing the flow from the fistula into PA.

necessary. However, double-umbrella devices are typically used for large fistulas and coils are used for small fistulas (Figure 1-51).

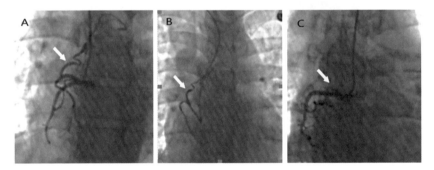

Figure 1-51　Comparison of ICA before and after interventional closure of RCA-PA fistula. A: CAF was found by ICA; B: RCA-PA fistula was found by superselective ICA; C: Angiographic changes after TCC.

The clinicians suggested that Amplatzer vascular plug provides one of the best TCC techniques due to the variety of available sizes, the ability to reposition after initial placement, and overall safety. Currently standard application criteria have been established for these vascular plugs (Figure 1-52). Since 2008, the use of Amplatzer vascular plug is popular and more common.

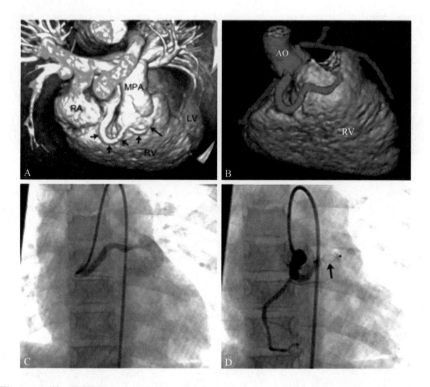

Figure 1-52 CCF between RCA and RV in a 9-month-old girl. A: CT showed the dilated conal branch (short arrows) draining into RVOT (long arrow); B: CT demonstrated the CCF and AO in red, and normal RCA and LCA in blue; C-D: Angiographic images (5 years later) confirmed the CCF (C), and an occluding device (arrow) was placed in the distal part of the fistula (D).

Balloon stent grafts are also popular in CAF closure techniques. Unfortunately, closure with these grafts is associated with a high risk of in-stent thrombosis or re-stenosis. Due to this, they are often indicated when CABG is part of the corrective regimen.

As with any surgical endeavor, surgical and transcatheter process of CAF have some risks including device embolization, arrhythmia, and AMI. Additionally, a case reported dead after catheter procedure for CAF was caused by a device that recoiled into LM. To avoid short- and long-term complications associated with TCC procedures, follow-up angiographic studies must be regularly performed. During follow-up, myocardial scintigraphy after transcatheter or surgical closure of CAF is also an important technique in order to recognize and/or avoid recanalization, AN formation, or AMI. The Texas Heart Institute reported a 2% overall mortality in surgical CAF closure. The majority of the deaths were associated with comorbidities, including cardiac lesions.

Wu YH reported a 7-month-old infant with giant and tortuous RCA-RA fistula and was successfully treated by TCC with Amplatzer duct occluder (Figures 1-53, 1-54).

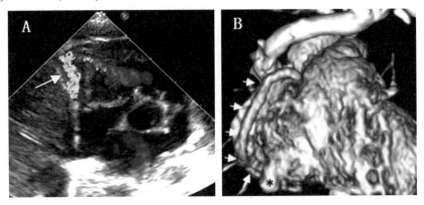

Figure 1-53   Echo showed dilated RCA (arrow in A); CT showed lageniform CAF (*) from RCA (arrows) to the inferior wall of RV (B).

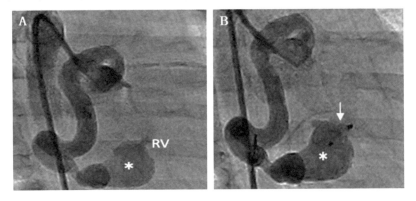

Figure 1-54   RCA angiogram revealed that the aneurysmal fistula (asterisks) had arisen from the distal RCA and drained into the inferior wall of RV. The shape of the fistula was lageniform. The aneurysmal tract of the fistula was 6 mm wide, and the narrowest diameter of the drainage site was 1.5 mm (A); Post-procedural RCA angiogram showed that the ADO Ⅱ device (arrows) occluded the fistula with minimal residual shunt, with one disk in the aneurysmal tract (B).

The piccolo occluder was originally designed for occlusion of PDA in premature newborns weighing more than 700 g. Materna O reported that it could be used off-label for the occlusion of CAF in a newborn (Figure 1-55).

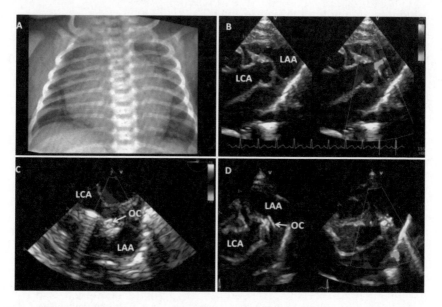

Figure 1-55 A left CAF was diagnosed prenatally at 22 weeks of gestation. An enlarged LCA was connected to LAA at the site of branching to LAD and LCX. The newborn (birthweight 2, 510 g) had a loud murmur, sinus tachycardia, and significant cardiomegaly (A). Echo confirmed the above-described anatomy (B). TCC of the fistula was indicated after 15 days due to persisting clinical signs of a significant shunt. Complete occlusion of the fistula and stable position of the occluder (OC) were confirmed on the following day by Echo (C & D).

Zhao X reported 26 patients with CAF for attempted combined therapy using coils and Onyx. In selected patients with CAF, this transcatheter embolization appears to be a valid option, providing a high success rate and low recanalization rate (Figures 1-56, 1-57).

Nair A reported a case of CAF with an unusually large fistulous sac within IVS. The fistula had connections with all the 3 major coronary arteries but did not have any exit resulting in to-and-fro blood flow within the sac and the feeding vessels. The patient was managed successfully by transcatheter coil embolization (Figure 1-58).

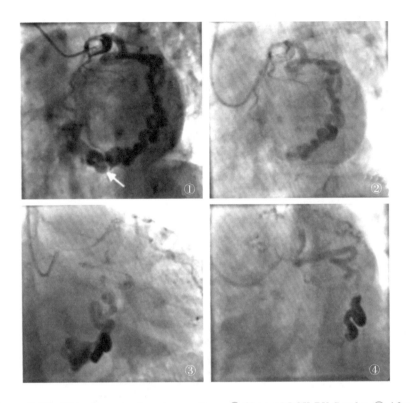

Figure 1-56   ICA of pre- and post-operation. ① Showed LCX-RV fistula; ② After 4 coils implanted; ③ After 6 coils implanted; ④ After Onyx-34 injected.

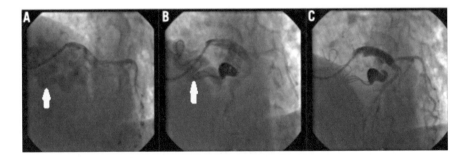

Figure 1-57   ICA of a giant fistula. A: A giant fistula (white arrow) originating from the LAD and draining into the PA was identified in a 63-year-old woman; B: 3 coils were initially deployed in the fistula, but significant residual flow remained (white arrow); C: Residual flow disappeared completely after injecting 0.6 ml of Onyx-34, as demonstrated by immediate post-embolization angiography.

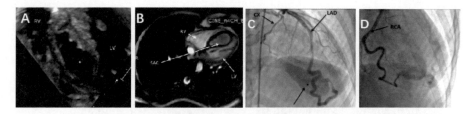

Figure 1-58   A: Echo showed the RV and LV with a fistulous sac (asterisk) burrowing IVS; B: MR showed the fistulous sac within IVS; C & D: ICA showed feeders into the sac (asterisk) from LAD, LCX and RCA.

Device migration is a known complication of TCC, for which surgical retrieval is required. In a study at the Mayo Clinic, only 2 of 99 patients developed migration, and the device was retrieved angiographically. Singh J reported a case with RCA-RVOT fistula, and device closure was performed with Amplatzer vascular plug. The device migrated to distal left PA and was retrieved after 8 years (Figures 1-59, 1-60).

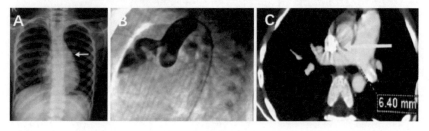

Figure 1-59   A: X-ray showed the device at a different position to the fistula site (yellow arrow); B: ICA showed a patent RCA-RVOT fistula; C: CT showed a hyperdense foreign body in the left PA 7 mm from its bifurcation (yellow arrow).

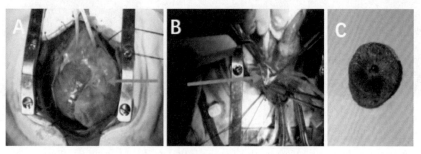

Figure 1-60   A: Operative photograph showed the patent fistula as an outpouching arising from RCA; B: The migrated device stuck in the left PA; C: The retrieved device.

13. Management

Luo L suggested that there is a potential for thrombotic events that may lead to AMI after CAF closure. Prophylactic low dose Aspirin or Indobufen is suggested in such cases. After PCI and/or atrial fibrillation, anticoagulant such as Warfarin, Rivaroxaban, or Dabigatran, is recommended. Angina secondary to CAF is managed according to the standard-of-care guidelines for CAD medical management. As such, β-blocker, calcium channel antagonist, nitrate, and Chinese herb may be prescribed. If additional medical intervention is used, regular follow-up must be performed to prevent new fistula, further dilation or residual shunt.

14. Patient education

This disease is relatively rare, with one of 50,000 CHD. The average age of initial symptoms was 43 years old. Patient education is very important because most people diagnosed with CAF have no symptoms. For other reasons, they are often accidentally informed of the existence of fistula during Echo or ICA. After diagnosis, it is essential to educate patients that CAF may develop symptoms after 20 years or less. Patients should be advised to pay attention to some relevant and possible symptoms, such as chest pain, exertional dyspnea, palpitation, and other cardiopulmonary symptoms. They should be informed of regular follow-up with clinicians and/or cardiologists. Once any of the above symptoms occur, they should be instructed to the nearest emergency room.

Patients who have received TCC or surgical repair of CAF should be encouraged to adhere to antiplatelet therapy (in some cases, anticoagulant) and follow-up closely with their cardiologists. The CAF patients should take more foods containing magnesium, chromium, zinc, calcium, selenium, and iodine. Foods rich in magnesium, such as millet, corn, bean products, medlar, and longan, can affect blood lipid metabolism and thrombosis, promote fibrinolysis, and prevent platelet aggregation. Trace chromium can prevent the formation of atherosclerosis and reduce cholesterol, and foods rich in chromium include yeast, beef, whole grain, cheese, brown sugar, etc. Foods containing more zinc, such as meat, oyster, egg, and milk, can also affect serum cholesterol content. Foods rich in calcium can prevent hypertension and hypercholesterolemia caused by a high-fat diet. Foods containing more selenium, such as oyster, fresh shellfish, shrimp, and barracuda, can resist atherosclerosis, reduce plasma viscosity, increase coronary blood flow, and reduce myocardial damage. Iodine can reduce the deposition of cholesterol on the blood vessel wall, and slow down or prevent the development of atherosclerosis. It is naturally beneficial to often eat seaweed, laver, and other seafood rich in iodine.

In addition, the CAF patients should take more protective food, such as onion, garlic, alfalfa, agaric, kelp, mushroom, and laver, because garlic and onion contain essential oil, an effective ingredient for preventing and treating atherosclerosis. Moderate tea drinking can also prevent and treat CAD because Chinese tea has the effect of anticoagulation and promoting fibrinolysis. Tea polyphenols can improve the permeability of microvascular wall, effectively enhance the elasticity and resistance of myocardial and vascular wall, and reduce the degree of atherosclerosis. Caffeine and theophylline can directly excite the heart, expand coronary arteries, and enhance myocardial function.

The diagnosis and treatment of CAF are highly dependent on an effective interprofessional team. For pediatric patient, caregiver must monitor the vital signs of newborn/infant to find any manifestations of shortness of breath and tachycardia. Neonatologist and pediatrician are essential to carefully identify any possible murmurs in infant patients, so refer these patients to a pediatric cardiologist.

For adult patients, resident and cardiologist should work together to correctly diagnose patients with CAF. These patients may have symptoms/signs of myocardial ischemia, CHF, or arrhythmia. Resident should complete appropriate preliminary examinations and consult with the cardiology team. Cardiologist can evaluate CAF, through Echo, CTA, or ICA, and radiologist need to read angiographic data properly. And then, based on the MDT results of cardiologist and thoracic surgeon, the doctor decided to apply TCC or surgical repair or conservative follow-up, but usually preferred non-invasive TCC first.

The key points of prevention:

(1) Prevent various possible pathogenic factors, vigorously promote eugenics and good parenthood, avoid virus infection in the early pregnancy, reduce the influence of adverse physical and chemical factors on the uterus, and carry out prenatal genetic or chromosome examination when necessary to prevent the disease.

(2) The treatment depends on the condition of the patient with CAF. Those with small shunt and no clinical symptoms may not need TCC or surgery, but IE should be prevented; those with symptoms generally advocate early TCC or surgery, including ligation or repair of the fistula, and closure with coil or occluder; for those who are not suitable for TCC and surgery for some reasons, drugs can be taken for symptomatic treatment.

15. Summary

CAF are anatomic abnormalities of the coronary artery but may be burdened by a number of complications if not detected and treated rapidly, especially if they are or become symptomatic. The suggested diagnostic approach is guided by the patient's symptoms, including the advanced imaging methods. If CAF is not incidental but symptomatic, mostly due to myocardial ischemia (angina, dyspnea, etc.), ICA is required in view of optimal therapeutic planning. Fistula management is variable and depends on several factors, including size and symptoms.

CAF, while rare, is pathophysiologically important and should be included in the differential diagnosis of cardiac-associated pathologies. Proper recognition, imaging, diagnosis, treatment, and symptom management can prevent potentially deadly cardiac complications associated with these anomalous communications.

According to the patient's symptoms, signs, Echo, MDCT scanning, and other imaging examinations, CAF can be preliminarily diagnosed. Selective

ICA can clearly show the shape, size, and location of CAF, which is the gold standard for diagnosing CAF. TCC of CAF is a minimally invasive, safe, and effective method, but indications must be strictly controlled. Surgical treatment can be selected for the followings: There are normal coronary artery branches near the fistula to be blocked; The fistula is seriously twisted; there are many outlets; TCC is difficult.

Chapter II Epidemiology

Highlights

- There are great differences in the incidence of CAF according to the different reports in clinical studies.

- CAF is rare, noted in $0.1\% - 0.2\%$ of ICA. A total of fewer than 400 papers had been reported by 1981, and about 400 papers by 2023.

- Previous studies have suggested that RCA-RV fistula is more common, but new research showed that the most common fistula is between LM or LAD and PA.

- Among all CAF, congenital is the first, acquired is the second, and the number is minimal. However, in ICA, the detection rate of various classifications and types differ.

- However, the outcome of clinically silent CAF found incidentally by Echo and CDE is unclear. In addition to individual health issues, the asymptomatic fistula mentioned in the Echo report and followed-up by Echo in a tertiary center carries psychological and economic burdens.

- The incidence of CAP is about $0.1\% - 0.58\%$; in coronary transluminal rotational atherectomy or laser angioplasty, the incidence is $0.5\% - 3.0\%$. In a few cases, CAP was not found during the operation, and a small amount of continuous bleeding led to pericardial tamponade dozens of minutes to hours after the operation. Timely diagnosis and active treatment are key to reducing the mortality of CAP.

However, CAF is an abnormal connection that connects one or more coronary arteries directly to heart chamber or major thoracic vessels without an interposed capillary bed. Fistulas that arise from a coronary artery and then terminate into the chamber of the heart are known as CCF, while those terminating into the vein are CAVF.

1. Epidemiology of congenital CAF

CAF's exact incidence is as yet unknown because the undiagnosed rate remains high, but it is estimated that the incidence of coronary anomalies is 0.2%-1.2% in the general population. CAF is present in 0.002% of the total population and represents about 0.2%-0.4% of all cardiac malformations and 14% of all CAA. Cheung DL and Gowda RM found that the detection rate of CAF in selective ICA was about 0.1%-0.2%, and the incidence in patients with CHF was about 0.08%-0.4%. Yamanaka O retrospectively analyzed the imaging data of 126,595 cases of ICA from 1960 to 1988, and found 1,686 patients (1.3%) with coronary malformation, 1,461 cases (87%) had abnormal origin of the coronary artery, and 225 cases (13%) had CAF (Table 2-1). Several studies report the presence of CAF in 0.3% of patients presenting with CHD, in 0.06% of children undergoing Echo, and in 0.13%-0.22% of adults undergoing ICA (Table 2-2).

Table 2-1 Incidence of congenital CAA (Yamanaka O, 1990)

	No	Incidence(%)	Anomalies(%)
Total ICA	126,595		
Total CAA	1,686	1.33	
Anomalies of origin and distribution	1,461	1.15	87
CAF	225	0.18	13

Table 2-2 Incidence of congenital CAF (Nakayama Y, 2010)

Author	Patients	CAF	Incidence(%)	Population
Gillebert 1986	14,708	20	0.13	Belgian
Yamanaka 1990	126,295	225	0.18	American
Bhandari 1993	4,486	8	0.11	Indian
Cebi 2008	18,272	10	0.05	German
Vavuranakis 1995	33,600	34	0.10	American
Nawa 1996	704	15	2.10	Japanese
Kardos 1997	7,694	5	0.06	Hungarian
Yildiz 2010	12,450	12	0.09	Turkish
Said 2006	30,829	51	0.16	Dutch
Chiu 2008	28,210	125	0.44	Chinese

Tian Y collected 945 patients who underwent coronary CTA in the hospital from 2010 to 2012. Taking ICA as the gold standard, just 2 cases of CAF were found. Zhu L retrospectively analyzed MPR, VR, MIP, and CPR images of 357 patients with CAA detected by coronary CTA, and found 1 case of CAF. Dai Q detected that LCA originated from PA in 4 cases (0.10‰) of 38,573 patients with CAA who completed MDCT; 12 cases (0.31‰) had multiple or large CAF. Cui M analyzed and compared the results of Echo, ICA, and surgery in 40 cases of congenital CAA. The results showed that the coronary artery originated from PA in 12 cases (30%); coronary artery originated from aortic sinus in 8 cases (20%); CAF occurred in 20 cases (50%). The sensitivity and specificity of Echo were 92% and 100%, respectively.

Ethnic group and gender do not affect the incidence of CAF, and multiple fistulas are present in 10.7%–16%, while single fistula is much more common, being present in 90% of all CAF cases.

Cai W retrospectively analyzed the angiographic data of 1,020 elderly patients aged ≥ 60 from 2000 to 2009. A total of 31 cases (3%) of CAA were detected, including 17 cases (54.8%) of abnormal origin and distribution of coronary artery, 9 cases (29%) of CAF, and 5 cases of abnormal coronary artery structure (16.2%). The authors believe that CAA in the elderly is not uncommon. ICA is one of the main methods to diagnose CAF in the elderly, but most CAF does not lead to serious clinical consequences.

Said SAM reported 2 typical cases of CAF at the age of 80 and discussed the relationship between gender and CAF after reviewing some previous studies (Figure 2-1). The authors believe that among the super-elderly patients, the incidence of CAF is higher in women than in men (70% vs. 30%), double CAF is more common in women (23% vs. 12%), there is no difference between men and women in the coronary artery-PA fistula (60% vs. 53%), the incidence of tumor-like dilatation is higher in women than in men (40% vs. 18%), 53% of women and 35% of men need surgery, and the incidence of tumor-like dilatation in Asian population is 65%, higher than

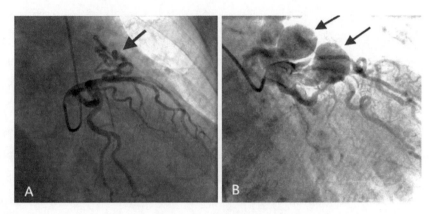

Figure 2-1 Angiographic findings of LCA-PA fistula in women around 80 years old. A: 70-year-old patient with tortuous LCA-PA fistula (arrow); B: In a 90-year-old patient with LCA-PA and AN, the size of AN was 52.5 ×48 mm and 51 mm ×48 mm (arrow), respectively.

16% of non-Asian people.

Much of the statistical data regarding the incidence, etiology, presentation, and treatment of CAF is derived from cohort data in retrospect and prospect, as well as numerous case reports. Alpert BS published an epidemiological investigation report in 1984. It was found that 92% of CAF communicated with the right cardiac system (RV, RA, and CS), and the fistula into RV accounted for the first (44%), followed by RA and PA. Few patients had drainage sites in the left cardiac system (most of them were fistula into LA). However, clinical observations over the past 3 decades have found that this incidence has changed and LAD-PA fistula may occupy the first place.

Up to 1980, 325 cases have been reported worldwide, accounting for 0.2% of congenital cardiovascular malformations. From 1980 to 2014, more than 3,000 therapeutic cases were reported at home and abroad, but the actual number of detected and treated cases was much higher than the number of reported cases. Morita H reported a case of giant AN with LAD-PA fistula, and reviewed the literature before 2012 (Figures 2-2, 2-3).

From 2014 to 2023, more than 800 rare or therapeutic cases were

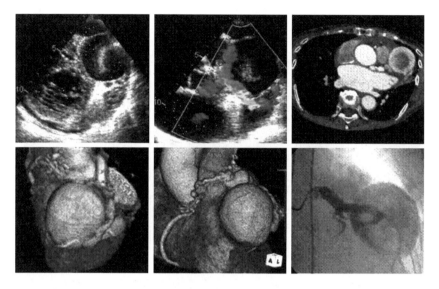

Figure 2-2   Imaging examination of giant AN with LAD-PA fistula.

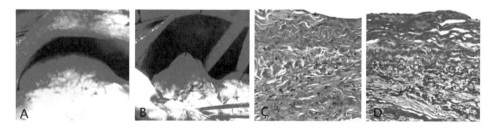

Figure 2-3   A & B: Surgical field of giant AN with LAD-PA fistula; C & D: Pathological changes of AN wall, lymphocyte aggregation (C) and connective tissue hyperplasia (D).

reported, and by 2023, there were more than 1,000 important international papers on CAF. ICA showed that the incidence of congenital CAF was 0.3%–0.8%, and the detection rate of Echo was 0.06%–0.2%, accounting for 0.2% of cardiac surgery in the same period.

Feng XQ found 47 cases of CAF in 12,032 angiographic patients, accounting for about 0.39%. Wang JN. retrospectively analyzed the imaging data of coronary CTA. The results showed that 11 coronary artery-pulmonary fistula (CAPF) cases were detected in 6,915 cases, and the detection rate was about 0.16%. Among them, 6 cases (54.55%) had RCA fistula into PA,

3 cases (27.27%) had LCA fistula into PA, and 2 cases (18.18%) had double CAF into PA (Figure 2-4).

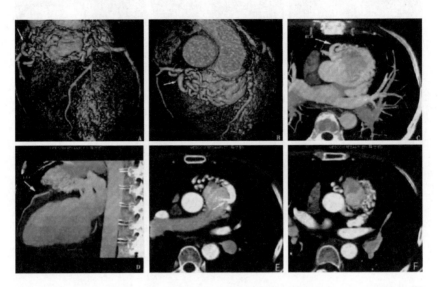

Figure 2-4 CT findings of double CAPF.

Allen KY and others retrospectively analyzed the clinical data of 100 heart transplant patients in 2 medical centers from 1999 to 2009. During the follow-up of 8.7 years (average 4.2 years), 52 cases of CAVF, 20 cases of CCF and 11 cases of mixing. 19 cases (19%) were multiple ACVF, and 52 patients had 77 outlets of fistula. 56% were small CAF, 36% were medium size and 8% were giant CAF. 95% of ACVF was found at the first ICA after heart transplantation (1 year after operation). Uechi Y, Remadi F, Delarche N, Lefevre T, Zhang GB and other scholars reported more than 200 cases of small CAF, and the clinical characteristics and treatment strategies of this type of patients were analyzed. Small CAF is not clinically detectable, generally asymptomatic, can close over time, and is not clearly associated with significant long-term complications. In almost 40% of the reviewed subjects with congenital coronary artery-ventricular MMF, T wave inversion was present in the precordial leads of the ECG in association with or without apical hypertrophic cardiomyopathy. For adult patients with congenital coronary artery-ventricular multiple micro-fistulas, conservative medical management is the treatment of choice. Limited data were reported on adult patients with solitary CCF. Within the entity of CCF, each subtype has its own specific characteristics such as origin, termination of fistulas, and treatment options. In addition, there were few reports on the implantation of an ICD in patients with extensive congenital MMF in association with syncope.

Although CAF is rare in the large category of CHD, it is a very common disease in the small category of CAA. ICA showed that congenital CAF accounts for about 50% of CAA in children, and the incidence of 1– 10 years old is the highest. Ying S, Tao W, Wang Y and others reported the younger cases of CAF (Figures 2-5, 2-6 and 2-7).

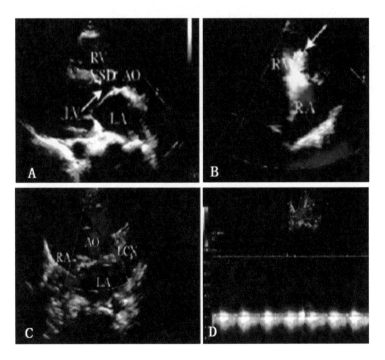

Figure 2-5   Echo findings of TOF with RCA-RV fistula (A & B) and LCX-RA (C & D) fistula.

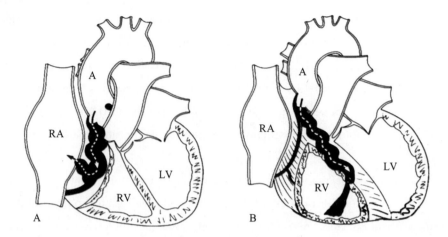

Figure 2-6　Diagrams of RCA-RA fistula (A) and coronary artery-RV fistula (B).

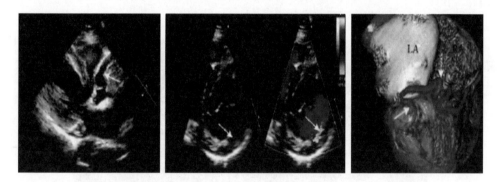

Figure 2-7　Echo and CT images of RCA-LV fistula.

　　In 1999, Yao M summarized the ICA data of 4,173 patients to determine various congenital CAA accurately. The results showed that 50 cases (1.2%) with abnormal origin of coronary artery were detected, including 42 cases (84.0%) had abnormal origin of coronary artery, 7 cases (14.0%) had abnormal origin of LCA, and 1 case (2.0%) had abnormal origin of both LCA and RCA. Twenty-eight cases (0.7%) of various types of CAF were detected, of which 18 cases (64.3%) were CAPF (Table 2-3). The authors believe that the clinical symptoms and signs of congenital CAF in adults are often atypical or absent, which are usually accidentally found in cardiac catheterization. ICA is the most important examination method to diagnose various types of CAF.

Table 2-3   Types of CAF in 28 cases

Type of CAF	Patients	Detection rate
LAD-PA fistula	10	
LCX-PA fistula	5	
RCA-PA fistula	1	
LCX-right PA fistula	1	
RCA-RV fistula	3	
RCA-small cardiac vein fistula	1	
LAD and RCA-PA fistula	1	
Total (coronary artery-right cardiac cavity and PA fistula)	22	0.53%
LAD-LV fistula	3	
LCX-LA fistula	1	
LAD and LCX-LV fistula	1	
RCA-LV fistula	1	
Total (coronary artery-left cardiac cavity fistula)	6	0.14%
Total	28	0.67%

Wu XS retrospectively analyzed coronary CTA and clinical data of patients with CAPF (Figure 2-8). The results showed that 23 cases (0.17%) of CAPF were detected in 13,387 cases, including 7 cases (30%) with single CAF and 16 cases (70%)with double CAF. All cases showed fistula vessels, and 6 cases showed localized tumor-like dilatation. Contrast agent staining was found in 19 cases of pulmonary artery trunk or jet sign.

Li J and others retrospectively analyzed the imaging data of 28 cases of adult CAPF diagnosed by coronary CTA (Figure 2-9): the origin, number, and course of fistula vessels (tubular dilatation or earthworm-like tortuous dilatation, mural sign); location, number, size and signs of CAPF (perforation sign, smoke sign, jet sign). The shape of tortuous dilation of fistula vessels include: tubular dilation in 7 cases, earthworm-like tortuous

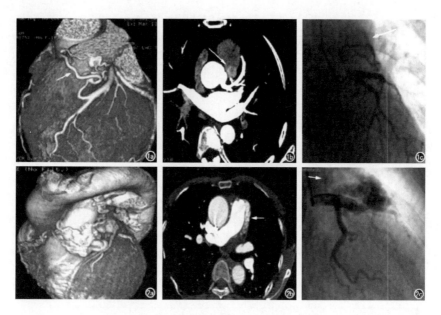

Figure 2-8   Imaging examination of CAPF.
1a-1c: One case; 2a-2c: Another case.

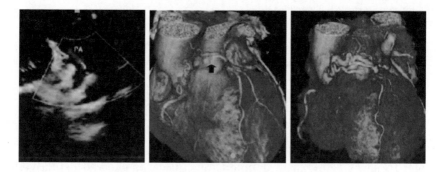

Figure 2-9   Echo and CT findings of CAPF.

dilation in 21 cases (9 cases with AN). Fistulas were located in the anterior wall of PA in 10 cases, the left wall in 17 cases, and the right wall at the bifurcation of PA in 1 case; the size of PA fistula is about 1.7–7.4 mm, with an average of about 3.3 mm. CT signs of PA fistula: 28 cases of perforating sign, 11 cases of jet sign or ejection sign, and 14 cases of smoke sign.

Zou J retrospectively analyzed the diagnostic value of 320 slice spiral CT in CAPF (Figure 2-10). Among the 5 cases of CAF, there was RCA-PA fistula in 2 cases, LCA-PA fistula in 2 cases, and double CAPF in 1 case. All images showed the relationship and location of abnormal vessels and PA through VR, MIP, CPR, and other reconstructed images.

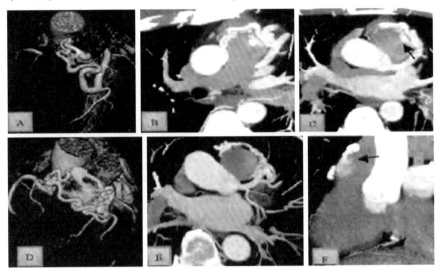

Figure 2-10   CT findings of LAD-PA fistula.
A-C: One patient; D-F: Another patient.

More than 80% of patients have CHF after the age of 20, especially after 40. The incidence of ischemic angina caused by coronary steal phenomenon is 6.7%–18.4%, but AMI is rare (3%). Although angina occasionally occurs in childhood, it often occurs after age 50. Li T reported a case of myocardial perfusion imaging of AMI caused by LAD-LV fistula (Figure 2-11).

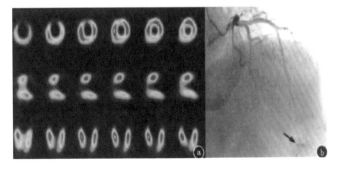

Figure 2-11   Myocardial perfusion imaging (a) and angiographic finding of LAD-LV fistula (b).

2. Epidemiology of acquired CAF

The incidence of CAP is 0.15%–2.5%, an infrequent complication of PCI. Most CAP are large vessel perforations and often require further intervention, but the incidence of death or emergent cardiac surgery is low.

Ellis SG collected 12,900 PCI cases from 11 heart centers in the United States, of which 62 patients had CAP (0.5%). Ellis classified CAP into 3 types, among which type II perforation was the most common (50%), followed by type III (25.8%) and type I (21%), and only a very few cases with contrast agent draining into atrium, ventricle or CS (3.2%). Type I perforation has the best prognosis. Generally, no special treatment is needed, and the risk of pericardial tamponade is 8%; sometimes, type II perforation only needs low-pressure balloon expansion to block the orifice, which can stop extravasation of contrast agent, and the risk of pericardial tamponade is 13%; type III perforation is the most dangerous, the risk of pericardial tamponade is 63%, the mortality is as high as 20%–44%, and 60% require emergent surgery. When the contrast agent extravasates into atrium, ventricle or CS, the prognosis is usually better (Table 2-4, Figures 2-12, 2-13).

Table 2-4　Types and manifestations of CAP

Type of CAP	Findings	Risk of cardiac tamponade
I	Contrast agent retention without overflow	8%
II	Pericardial or myocardial staining (overflow), no ejection	13%
III A	The contrast agent is sprayed into the whole pericardial cavity through an open port > 1 mm	63%
III B, Intracavitary perforation	CAP into anatomical cavity, such as CS	–

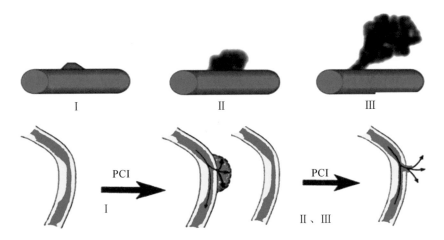

Figure 2-12　Schematic diagram of Eillis classification of CAP.

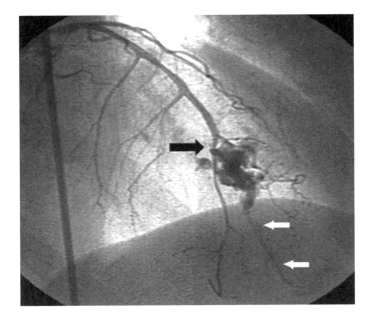

Figure 2-13　Angiographic finding of Ellis Ⅲ CAP. Type Ⅲ perforation in the middle and distal LAD (black arrow), the contrast agent jet penetrated into the pericardial cavity. After the perfusion balloon was placed, the contrast agent still continued to penetrate into the pericardial cavity and led to pericardial tamponade. After pericardial puncture and drainage, the patient was sent to the operating-room for emergent surgery.

In addition to Ellis classiffication, there are some alternative taxonomy of CAP.

Fukutomi type I : The contrast agent leaks to the epicardium without a jet of contrast extravasation; Type II : The contrast agent leaks to the epicardium with a jet of contrast extravasation.

Kini type I : The contrast agent leaks to the myocardium, but there is no jet leakage; Type II : Obvious leakage of contrast agent into pericardium, CS and cardiac cavity.

Ajluni type I : The contrast agent exudes from the blood vessel in mushroom shape or the contrast agent extravasate; Type II : Continuous leakage of contrast agent into pericardium, cardiac cavity or CS.

The perforation caused by balloon, guidewire, and other uncertain factors accounted for 74% , 20% and 6% , respectively. The incidence of death after perforation is about 0%–9.5% , AMI is 4%–26% , and emergent surgery is 24%–36% . It can occur in vessels of different sizes, mostly in the branches and peripheral vessels. It can be obvious leakage or local hematoma, which shows that the contrast agent leaks directly into the pericardium or local area, or it can be a small leakage that is not easy to be found.

Patients with type I and type II (Fukutomi classification) perforations were managed by observation only (35% and 0% , respectively), reversal of anticoagulation (57% and 94%), pericardiocentesis and drainage (27% and 61%), and prolonged perfusion balloon angioplasty (16% and 100%). Two patients with type II perforations required emergent CABG. There were no in-hospital deaths. Late pseudoaneurysms developed in 18 (28.6%) patients during the 13 months' follow-up period, and were more common in patients with type II perforations (72.2% vs 11.1% with type I perforations; p < 0.001). During the follow-up period, no patient had evidence of coronary rupture. The results suggest that CAP after PCI can be managed without cardiac surgery in the majority of cases. Late pseudoaneurysms developed in some patients, particularly in patients with type II perforations, but there were no late consequences of CAP.

Avula V examined the clinical, ICA, procedural characteristics, management, and outcomes of CAP at a tertiary care institution. Between 2014 and 2019, perforation occurred in 70 case of 10, 278 PCI (0.7%). Patient age was 71±12 years, 66% were men, and 30% had prior CABG. Among perforation cases, the prevalence of CTO was 33%, moderate/severe calcification was 66%, and moderate/severe tortuosity was 41%. The frequency of Ellis class Ⅰ, Ⅱ, and Ⅲ perforations were 14%, 50%, and 36%, respectively. Most (73%) were large vessel perforations, 16 (23%) were distal vessel perforations, and 3 (4%) were collateral vessel perforations. Hypotension occurred in 26%, pericardial effusion in 36%, and tamponade in 13%; 47% of perforations did not have clinical consequences. Perforations were most often treated with prolonged balloon inflation (63%), reversal of anticoagulation (39%), and covered stent implantation (33%); the success rates of technical and procedural were 73% and 60%, respectively; major periprocedural adverse cardiac events occurred in 21% of the patients; 3 patients (4%) required emergent CABG and 4 (6%) died.

CAP is a rare but potentially life-threatening complication of PCI, however, if recognized and managed promptly, its adverse consequences can be minimized. Risk factors for CAP include the use of advanced PCI technique (such as atherectomy, and CTO interventions) and treatment of severely calcified lesions. There are 3 major types of CAP depending on location: (a) large vessel perforation, (b) distal vessel perforation, and (c) collateral perforation. Large vessel perforation is usually treated with implantation of a covered stent, whereas distal and collateral vessel perforations are usually treated with coil or fat embolization.

With increasing PCI volumes and complexity of CTO, the incidence of CAP is likely to rise. Adherence to good catheterization laboratory practices, availability of dedicated equipment to seal CAP, the perform of pericardiocentesis, and sufficient hemodynamic support, as well as adequate training, are pillars for the prevention and optimal management of CAP during CTO intervention.

Chapter Ⅲ　Etiology

Highlights

- Congenital CAF is still the first, but with the development of medical technology and the subsequent complications of various operations, the incidence of acquired CAF is also increasing.

- In the early stage of pregnancy, the risk factors (RF) of fetal CAF included the mother being infected by rubella and other viruses, being undernourished, the uterus being affected by physical and chemical (radiation, drugs, etc.) and genetic factors.

- Prevent various possible pathogenic factors of CAF and vigorously promote eugenics. In the early stage of pregnancy, the women should avoid viral infection, reduce the influence of adverse physical and chemical factors on the uterus, and carry out prenatal gene spectrum or chromosome examination if necessary.

- Cardiovascular diseases, such as CAD, vasculitis, IE, and others, can cause the damage of the coronary artery and the adhesion surrounding cardiac cavity or large blood vessels, and finally result in acquired CAF.

- Trauma is the main cause of acquired CAF, especially penetrating injuries, such as knife stabbing injury, gunshot wound, steel and glass debris flying injury. Blunt chest trauma can also lead to CAF.

Although in the past, CAF was usually congenital, over the years, the development and dissemination of interventional and surgical techniques have resulted in a change in its etiology, with a higher prevalence of acquired CAF, which may include those secondary to IE, aortic dissection, previous surgery, endomyocardial biopsy, coronary angioplasty and bypass surgery, valve replacement, cardiac transplantation, trauma, permanent pacemaker implantation, ablation of accessory pathway, neoplasm, and iatrogenic management of Kawasaki disease (Table 3-1, Figure 3-1).

Table 3-1   Etiology of CAF

A. Congenital
1. Embroyonic
2. Multiple; systemic hemangioma

B. Acquired
1. Closed-chest ablation of accessory pathway
2. PCI
3. Hypertrophic cardiomyopathy
4. Right/left ventricular septal myectomy
5. Penetrating and nonpenetrating trauma
6. AMI
7. Dilated cardiomyopathy
8. Mitral valve surgery
9. "Sign" of mural thrombus
10. Tumor
11. Permanent pacemaker placement
12. Cardiac transplantation
13. Endomyocardial biopsy
14. CABG

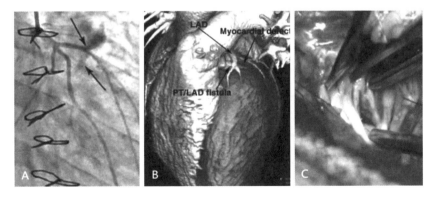

Figure 3-1   Angiogram (A), CT image (B), and surgical field (C) of traumatic LAD-PA fistula

1. Etiology of congenital CAF

From the embryological point of view, the congenital CAF is due to the persistence of intramyocardial trabecular connections formed by endothelial cells and blood lacuna that are formed initially within the cardiac venous plexus and subsequently with the epicardial coronary arteries (Figures 3-2, 3-3).

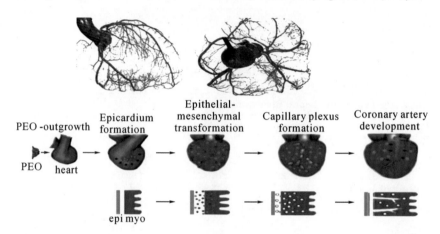

Figure 3-2　Vascular network of distal branches of coronary artery and development of coronary arteries. Movement of the proepicardial organ (PEO) to and over the heart is shown in the top panel, and mesenchymal migration and differentiation are shown in the bottom panel. The PEO (blue) is seen as an outgrowth from the dorsal body wall that moves to the looping heart (red). Next, migrating epithelium is seen spreading over the heart. In cross section, the epithelium is seen as a single cell layer. Epithelial/mesenchymal transition provides cells that migrate into the myocardium. Vasculogenic cells differentiate and link to form plexus that induce other mesenchymal cells to become smooth muscle. These plexus are remodeled into definitive arteries, and the most proximal points of the major coronaries finally link up with the aorta.

Branton H found the deletion of 22q11.2 gene fragment in a child with LV noncompaction and CAF. Delgado A reported an AMI case of hypertrophic cardiomyopathy, LV noncompaction with CAF (Figure 3-4), and the proposition of whether these 3 genetic diseases belong to the same genotype is put forward. Ann N found that CAF may be related to the loss of Gpc3 function (Figure 3-5).

The research of Zhou B and others revealed the new origin of coronary artery vessels-endocardium for the first time by using genetic pedigree tracing

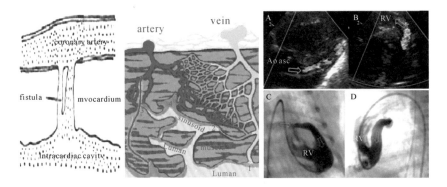

Figure 3-3   Schematic diagram of the formation of congenital CAF and a female neonate with LCA-RV fistula.

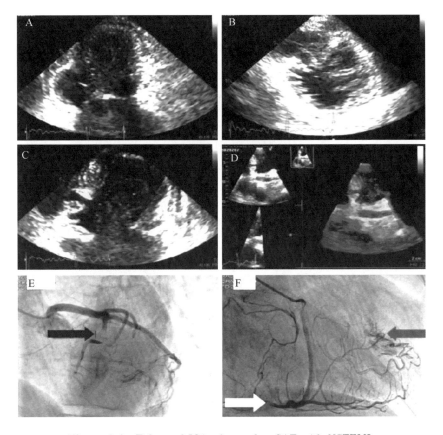

Figure 3-4   Echo and ICA of complex CAF with NSTEMI.

A   B

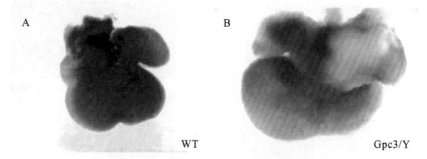

WT   Gpc3/Y

Figure 3-5 Decreased Shh mRNA levels in Gpc3 deficient heart.

technology (Figure 3-6). This significant discovery has laid a theoretical foundation for the clinical angio-regenerative treatment of AMI and the study in vitro artificial heart angiogenesis. The authors believe that this endogenous mechanism of rapid postnatal coronary artery growth provides important clues for exploring the pathogenesis, diagnosis, and treatment of CHD, such as myocardial insufficiency and congenital CAF.

  Hiroshi K reported the first case of CAF with aneurysmal change in a patient with immunoglobulin G4-related disease (IgG4-RD). In patients with IgG4-RD, vasculature is commonly affected with the abdominal aorta as the

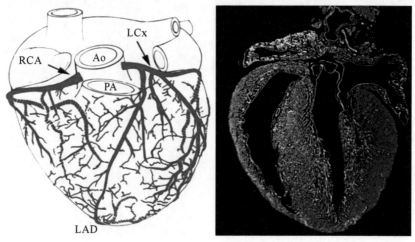

Figure 3-6 Schematic diagram of endocardial origin theory of coronary artery vessels.

most common site of cardiovascular lesions. Aortic abnormalities comprise some of the pathophysiological effects of IgG4-RD, and a possible role of atherosclerotic plaque in the pathogenesis of IgG4-related periaortitis has been suggested. Similar mechanisms may affect the coronary arteries in patients with IgG4-RD. The pericardium also can be affected by IgG4-RD. Like the retroperitoneal space, closed cavity spaces are preferred lesion sites for IgG4-RD. In this case, the author also observed circumferential mural thickening of LAD, pericardial nodular inflammation, and AN of CAPF (Figure 3-7). Each of these features was located close to the thickened pericardium. These lesions might result from inflammation of the pericardial space, which extended to the coronary pulmonary artery vessels. This case will enhance our understanding of the pathological mechanisms of IgG4-RD inflammation (Figure 3-8).

The animal experiments of Kim AJ and others found that CT has important diagnostic value for small CAF, small orifice, and fistula with abnormal tortuosity (Figure 3-9).

Tomohiro I reported a case with Kawasaki disease and CAPF. Although

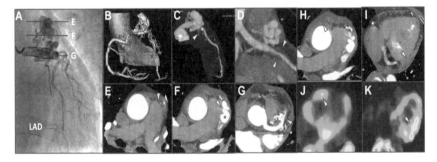

Figure 3-7   LAD-PA fistula was acquired by ICA (A). CT scan (B-G) and PET/CT are lined up in each corresponding slice (H-K). Arrowhead in (C) indicated calcified plaque and 50% stenosis of the proximal LAD. Detailed analysis of ICA and CT scan images revealed no other atherosclerotic changes. Arrowhead in (D) indicated circumferential mural thickening of LAD. Axial imaging of CT scan demonstrated inflow and outflow of fistula in each corresponding slice (E-G). The fistula had a single inflow from LAD and double outflow to the left PA (E-G). The red star in (F) showed AN. The area of thickened pericardium corresponded to the lesion revealed on PET/CT with increased uptake (arrowhead in H-K).

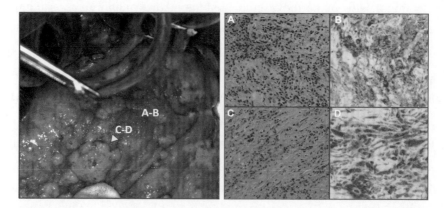

Figure 3-8　Numerous white nodules (yellow arrowhead) were observed on the surface of RV, with some surrounding the fistula (blue arrowhead). Histopathological investigation of the resected CAPF and AN (A-B) and the resected white nodule located on the surface of pericardium (C-D). A: Massive lymphoplasmacytic infiltrates were shown mainly in the adventitia side to the middle layer of the vasculature, as demonstrated by hematoxylineeosin staining; B: Immunohistological analysis using an anti-IgG4 antibody revealed that most of the infiltrated cells were IgG4-positive plasma cells with IgG4/IgG ratio of 40% to 80%; C: Lymphoplasmacytic infiltrate was observed within the fibroelastic tissue; D: Immunohistological analysis using an anti-IgG4 antibody revealed that most infiltrated cells were IgG4-positive plasma cells with IgG4/IgG ratio greater than 80%.

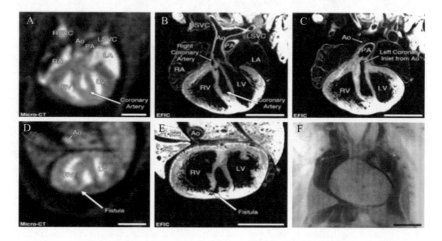

Figure 3-9　CT examination of CAF in newborn rat.

no coronary artery lesion had been found at the acute phase, aneurysmal dilation tends to progress readily when CAPF is located in the proximal part (Figures 3-10, 3-11). Because AN diameter is small and the patient is asymptomatic, restriction of most vigorous exercise and prevention of IE are recommended.

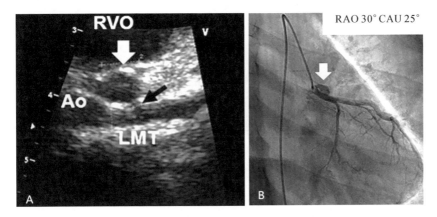

Figure 3-10   A: Echo showed AN (white arrow) located in the front of LM, communicating with PA through a narrow channel (black arrow); B: ICA showed AN (white arrow). LMT: left main trunk; RVO: right ventricular outflow tract.

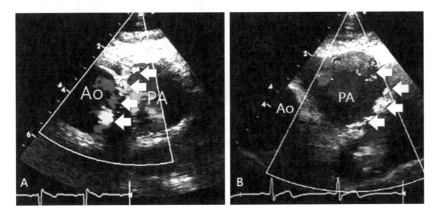

Figure 3-11   Echo showed blood flow of CAPF (white arrows). A: A fistula streams to the medial side of PA; B: Another fistula streams to the lateral side of PA.

Masaru Y demonstrated Kugel's artery-CS fistula in a 71-year-old female presenting with mitral valve regurgitation. MDCT enabled us to identify the precise course of this artery, especially its spatial relationship with cardiac structures (Figures 3-12, 3-13).

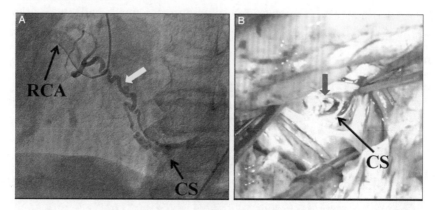

Figure 3-12 Angiogram demonstrated a tortuous CAVF (arrow in A) which originated from the proximal RCA and drained into CS. At surgery, this CAVF was identified on the roof of RA, and its drainage site was found in CS (arrow in B).

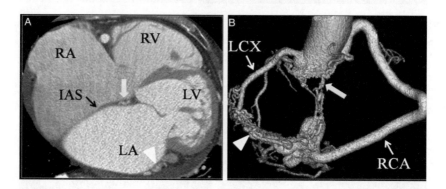

Figure 3-13 MDCT showed CAVF originated from the proximal RCA, ran posteriorly on RA wall, entered the interatrial septum (arrow in A and B), ran towards the crux of the heart, and finally drained to CS. Thus, the author confirmed this CAVF to be Kugel's artery. Another CAVF between LCX and CS was also demonstrated (arrow head). CAVF including Kugel's artery was ligated. In the present case, ICA was able to show CAVF from RCA, but failed to demonstrate the precise course. On the other hand, MDCT demonstrated the precise course of this CAVF, especially in its spatial relation to cardiac structures. IAS: interatrial septum.

Zhao L described a rare case of fetal CAF draining into LV using cross-sectional and CDFI (Figures 3-14, 3-15, and 3-16). Simona L reported a

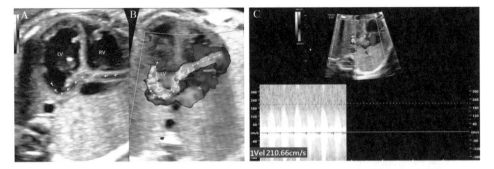

Figure 3-14 Identification of the course and outlet of CAF in a fetus of 24 gestational weeks. A tubular structure was visualized at the atrioventricular annulus when scanning a nonstandard four-chamber view (A). CDFI showed an abnormal flow from right to left draining into LV at the left side of atrioventricular annulus (B). Continuous wave Doppler showed a high-velocity blood pattern at the outlet of the fistula (C). The course of the abnormal blood flow with direction is indicated by the arrows.

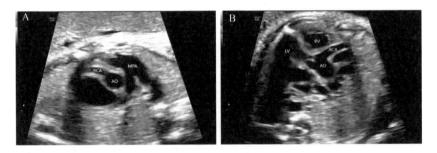

Figure 3-15 Identification of the origin of CAF. The dilatation of RCA with its origin from right aortic sinus was demonstrated when scanning aortic root short-axis view (A) and LVOT view (B), respectively.

female infant with Down's syndrome born at 37 weeks' gestation in good condition and discharged asymptomatic on the third day. Prenatal Echo at 22 weeks' gestation suggested a diagnosis of ASD and atrial septal aneurysm. Cardiological examination at 1 week of life revealed a grade 2/6 continuous murmur. Echo showed a large subaortic VSD, moderate tricuspid regurgitation, and CAF originating from an aneurysmal LM (Figure 3-17).

According to the drainage site of fistula, the possible cause of embryology is that under normal circumstances, there is a large sinus space in the embryonic myocardium. In the early stage of fetal development, these

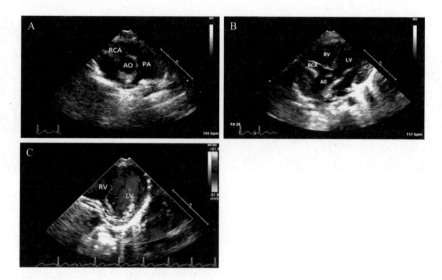

Figure 3-16 Identification of RCA-LV fistula in the same patient after birth. The dilatation of RCA with its origin from right aortic sinus was determined (A & B). CDFI showed an abnormal flow from right to left (indicated by the arrows), draining into LV at the left side of atrioventricular annulus (C).

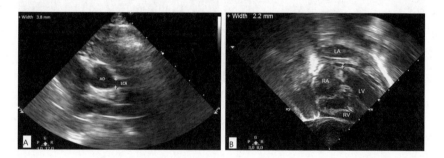

Figure 3-17 A: Echo showed the dilated LCA as wide as 3.8 mm; B: Subcostal four-chamber view showed a fistula (2.2 mm wide) that originates from LM.

sinusoids freely interact with the cardiac cavity and develop coronary arteries, veins, and some venous plexus. With the continuous development of myocardium, the extensive connection between sinus space and vein, the arterial system gradually decreases. The sinusoidal spaces in the myocardium are compressed into a network of capillaries. The outermost almost completely disappeared, while the innermost capillary network remained and communicated with the cardiac cavity. For some reason, the development of the local area of the embryonic myocardium stops in the early stage, and the sinus space persists, which constitutes CAF. Steinberg BL. and others believe that the primitive septum is not fully developed, and the coronary artery originates from PA, which makes the blood flow from coronary artery of high-pressure to PA of low-pressure and becomes the abnormal connection between coronary artery and PA. Awasthy N reported a special case of CAPF and pulmonary circulation dependent on coronary artery (Figure 3-18).

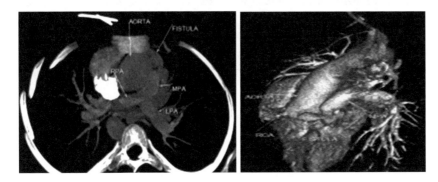

Figure 3-18   CT image of CAPF.

Mo H found 4 fetuses with CAF by Echo, and further confirmed this diagnosis by Echo and cardiac catheterization after birth (Figures 3-19, 3-20).

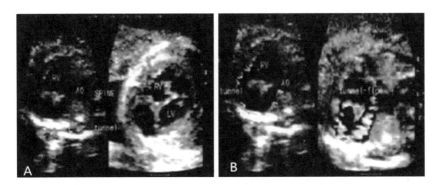

Figure 3-19   Echo findings of LCA-RV fistula.
A: Aneurysmal dilated coronary artery; B: Blood flow diagram.

Steinberg BL also believes that congenital AN is the cause of CAF. To explain this reason, the scholars cited 2 cases in the literature: one case of coronary artery had 17 AN of different sizes, with the largest diameter of

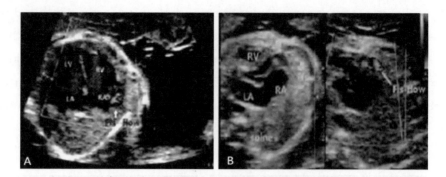

Figure 3-20   Echo findings of RCA-RV fistula.
A: Abnormal fistula (arrow); B: Blood flow diagram (arrow).

10 cm, but the fistula communicating with PA was only 2 mm; the diameter of the coronary artery AN in the other case was 23 cm, and the fistula drained into RA was also 2 mm. He believes that such a large AN cannot be caused by small CAF, but a congenital AN.

Perloff JK combined with literature reports and pointed out that the vessels of CAF often have cystic AN, which can reach a great extent. This kind of AN is believed to be secondary to fistula, rather than an independent congenital vascular malformation (Figure 3-21). This view is confirmed by the huge and tortuous RCA in traumatic coronary artery-RA fistula. Therefore, it is doubtful that primary AN is a cause of congenital CAF.

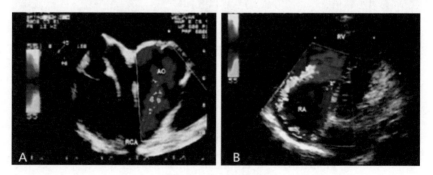

Figure 3-21   Echo examination of RCA-RA fistula.
A: TEE showed RCA aneurysmal dilatation and tortuous course; B: TTE showed RA turbulence spectrum.

Most CAF is simple/single (without other CHD), and a few are complex/complicated (with other CHD). Li S and Zheng M reported 2 cases of congenital RCA-LV combined with giant AN and aortic insufficiency (Figure 3-22).

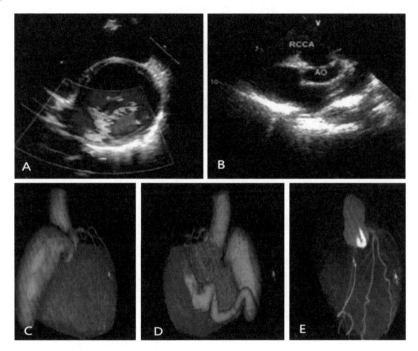

Figure 3-22   Echo and CT images of RCA-LV fistula.
A & B: One patient; C-E: Another patient with AN.

Liu MX Reported a 64-year-old woman presented with chest tightness, increased heart rate, and an elevated N-proBNP. Coronary CTA with cinematic rendering showed a 4.2 cm × 3.3 cm × 2.8 cm coronary artery-LA fistula. At ICA, numerous tiny feeding arteries were identified, along with 12 draining veins into LA (Figure 3-23).

Piskin F reported an extremely rare CAF extending from the sinoatrial nodal artery to RA (Figure 3-24).

Chen YH found that the course of coronary-bronchial artery fistula (CBF) usually was relatively fixed. The proportions of CBF originating from LCX, RCA, and LAD were 75%, 16.7%, and 8.3%, respectively. Preliminarily analysis of the correlation between the trend of CBF and the

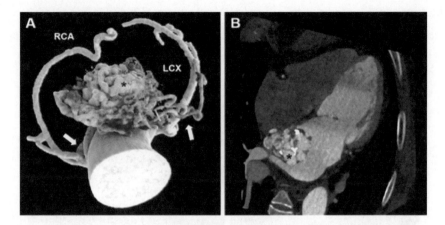

Figure 3-23 Cinematic rendering (A) and four-chamber CT image (B) depicted the fistula (asterisks) as a cauliflower-like mass with multiple calcified septa, sinuses, and double origins (white arrows) from both RCA and LCX to the fistula, which drains into the enlarged LA.

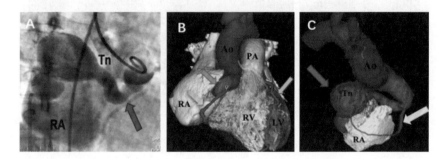

Figure 3-24 A: Selective ICA revealed the tunnel (blue arrow) draining into the RA; B: The volume rendering image revealed RCA (yellow arrow) separating from the tunnel (blue arrow) and following the posterior atrioventricular sulcus. LCA was shown to be normal (green arrow); C: The right atrial appendix subtracted from the volume rendering images, allowing the visualization of the entire tunnel, RA, and the fistula.

pulmonary diseases severity score showed that CBF was more likely to communicate with a bronchial artery on the side with a higher severity score. CBF may occur in patients with chronic pulmonary disease and hemoptysis, and its origin, course, and trend are characteristic. Detailed and comprehensive CTA analysis is helpful in improving the clinical treatment of hemoptysis with CBF (Figure 3-25).

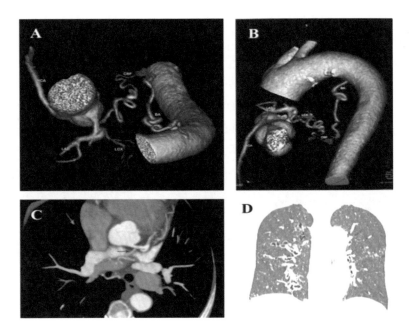

Figure 3-25   A 65-year-old female patient had cough and hemoptysis for 2 days. A & B: Showed the origin, morphology, course and spatial relationship between CBF and bronchial artery; C: Showed that CBF (black arrow) originated from the proximal LCX, ran in the transverse sinus and passed through the refection of the serous pericardium at the top of the LA into the mediastinum; D: Showed scattered multiple bronchiectases in the right lung and a few in the left lung.

Peng YX found the NEXN-truncated variant, NEXN-G100X, was associated with the development of coronary arteries and congenital CAA (Figure 3-26).

2. Etiology of CAP and others

CAP was common in the process of PCI 20 years ago, and now is rare, with an incidence of 0.19%–0.59% ; The mortality related to CAP can be as high as 7%–17% . The causes and RF of CAP include pathological, instrument, and technical factors. The pathological factors include chronic occlusive lesion, calcified lesion, severe distortion, and angulated lesion; the instrument factors include the improper use of guidewire, balloon and stent, as well as the use of special technologies such as cutting balloon, rotational atherectomy, and laser angioplasty; the technical factors are

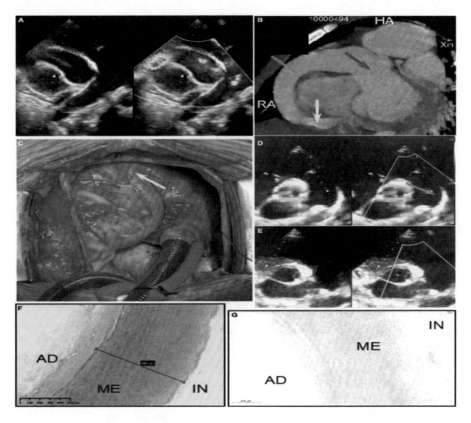

Figure 3-26　A & B: Showed RCA fistula by Echo and CT, respectively; C: Showed the intra-operative photograph of RCA fistula. The red arrow showed dilated ostium of RCA, and the green arrow showed the dilated main stem of RCA. The yellow arrow showed the fistula, and the blue arrow showed the coronary PDA; D & E: Showed Echo of coronary PDA before and after surgery, respectively; F: Showed the HE staining of the excised coronary artery aneurysm. The structure of the coronary artery is almost normal; G: Showed the negative calcium slats accumulation by Alizarin red staining of the excised coronary artery aneurysm. IN: intima; ME: media; AD: adventitia.

mainly caused by the inexperience of the operator, wrong choice of equipment, and insufficient judgment of the involved coronary arteries (Table 3-2).

Table 3-2   The RF of CAP

Patient related RF	Operator related RF	Instrument related RF
Female	Improper operation of guiding catheter	Hydrophilic coating guidewire
Elderly	Inexperience of the operator	Strong hardness guidewire
Old myocardial infarction	Excessive stent or balloon	Cutting balloon
Calcification	Excessive release pressure	New instruments (rotational atherectomy, laser angioplasty, etc.)
Angulation, tortuosity, long lesion	The head end of the guidewire is located at the extreme distal end of the blood vessel	IVUS catheter placed in false lumen of blood vessel
CTO		Others (ablation electrode, pacemaker, FFR, OCT, LAA occluder, etc.)
Myocardial bridge		

It is more common in complex PCI, such as CTO (4%), especially with retrograde approach (15%), unprotected left main PCI (0.9%), bypass graft PCI (0.32%–0.68%), and PCI in women and the elderly.

CAP is best classified according to its location into 3 categories: large vessel, distal vessel, or septal or epicardial collateral perforation. Each type has different risk factors and treatments. Common causes of large vessel perforation include use of oversized balloons and stents, use of high inflation pressures, particularly in tight, highly calcified lesions that are not properly remodeled by rotational atherectomy upfront. Furthermore, the aggressive plaque modification devices, such as cutting balloons, excimer laser, rotational, or orbital atherectomy devices, might increase the risk. In addition, rupture of inflated balloon or "grenadoplasty" may cause coronary perforation. Despite the fact that coronary intravascular lithotripsy shows a great success in remodeling calcified lesions, it might also increase the risk of large vessel CAP.

Distal vessel perforation is usually caused by distal wire migration, especially when polymer-jacketed guidewires are used. In one registry approximately 90% of distal wire induced CAP was due to the polymer-jacketed wire family.

Epicardial vessel collaterals perforation is not uncommon in retrograde approach for CTO PCI. Indeed, coronary perforation exists in 15% of total retrograde cases.

Interventional cardiologists should be able to recognize CAP and become familiar with available general and specific treatment options, as if recognized quickly and managed adequately, its adverse impact can be minimized. In general, proximal large vessel CAP usually require covered stents and distal or collateral vessel CAP can be safely treated with embolization therapy.

(1) CAP related to guidewire often occurs when using hydrophilic coating or guidewire with medium and above hardness to operate eccentric, bifurcated or occluded lesions;

(2) CAP is often related to balloon size or pressure, and often occurs in eccentric and calcified lesions;

(3) IVUS research found that stent related CAP is often seen in eccentric and calcified lesions. The pressure of stent release or balloon expansion is uneven for plaque and vascular wall, and the reaction force of stent to the hard plaque acts on the thinner vascular wall, resulting in vascular wall perforation.

Of course, in addition to CAP caused by the interventional procedure, other surgical operations, traumas and diseases can also cause perforation. Faustino A reported a case of secondary LCA-PA and LCA-SVC fistula (Figure 3-27). This is a 77-year-old patient who had undergone aortic valve replacement and was hospitalized due to dyspnea on exertion. Wei J and other scholars believe that the incidence of CAF has increased with the development of heart transplantation (Figure 3-28).

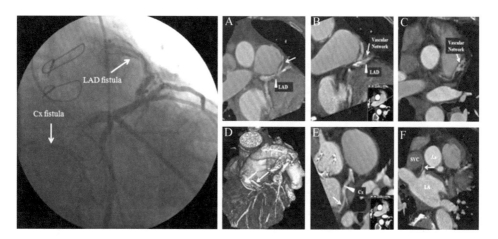

Figure 3-27   Imaging examination of secondary LAD-PA and LCX-SVC fistula.

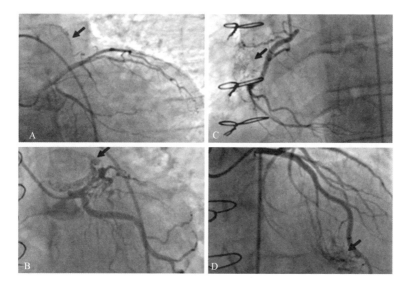

Figure 3-28   Formation of CAF after heart transplantation. A & B: 2 cases of LAD-PA fistula; C: RCA neovascularization, but not into RA; D: LAD-RV fistula was formed after myocardial biopsy.

The prognosis of CAP is related to the early diagnosis and treatment. Therefore, early recognition is significant for interventional doctors. CAP can lead to serious acute cardiac tamponade and even death. Therefore, preventing CAP is very important for every interventional physician and patient.

(1) Identify from the symptoms: The common complaints are sudden chest pain, chest tightness or palpitation, dyspnea and dizziness, and atypical symptoms are irritability, nausea, cold sweat, etc.

(2) Identify from the signs: Due to the rapid leakage of blood into the pericardial cavity, resulting in acute cardiac tamponade, which often causes serious hemodynamic disorders, sudden drop of systolic Bp (< 90 mmHg), jugular vein distention, distant heart sound, pale face, wet and cold skin, rapid and then slow heart rate, azygos pulse, and elevated central venous pressure. Some patients may have cardiac arrest.

(3) Identify from auxiliary examination: Echo is the gold standard for the diagnosis of pericardial effusion; Chest X-ray is a crucial method to confirm pericardial effusion for the cardiologist during PCI.

(4) Identify from ICA: The first manifestation is the extravasation of the contrast agent. The ICA findings show that the contrast agent exudes from the involved vessel and remains in the pericardial cavity, which is confirmed to be CAP.

During the operation, doctors should focus on the lesion but care more about the patient, and should focus on the guidewire and catheter, but pay more attention to the patient's Bp and heart rate. Two points are obvious. First, the patient's life is more important than his disease; second, the patient's condition, invasive pressure, ECG and blood oxygen saturation are the guarantee of interventional surgery.

During PCI, the results of each angiogram should be carefully observed to find small and distal perforation that is easy to be ignored. For patients prone to CAP during operation, Ⅱb/Ⅲa antagonists should be stopped after the operation to prevent the perforation caused by the guidewire and delayed cardiac tamponade after PCI. In order to prevent acute thrombosis in stents, dual antiplatelet therapy should not be discontinued. Ge L reported a series of cases of successful emergent treatment of CAP (Figure 3-29, 3-30).

Rodriguez MJ reported a case with late-acquired multiple CAF secondary to stab wound, diagnosed in the setting of ischemic heart failure secondary to

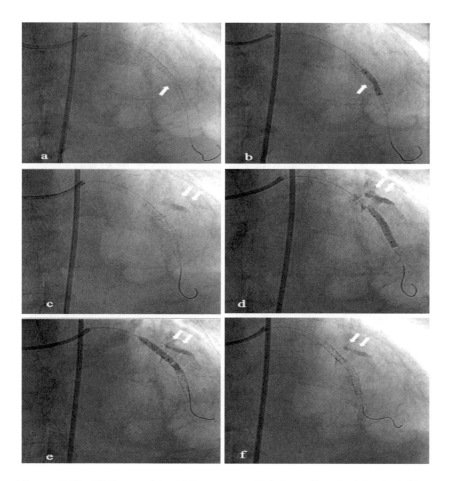

Figure 3-29 CAP caused by high-pressure dilatation after stent implantation. a: For occlusive lesions of LAD, after 2 drug-eluting stents (3.0 mm and 2.5 mm in diameter respectively) were placed in series, 40% of the residual stenosis was found at the tandem position of 2 stents (arrow); b: 3.0 mm non-compliance balloon posterior dilatation (18 atm); c: Vascular perforation, Ellis type Ⅲ (arrow); d & e: The balloon was filled with low pressure for a long time, but the contrast agent still exuded, so the JoMed PTFE covered stent was placed; f: Contrast agent exudation was terminated.

coronary steal syndrome (Figure 3-31).

Wang X reported a case of coronary artery—left atrial appendage (LAA) fistula caused by LAA occlusion (Figure 3-32).

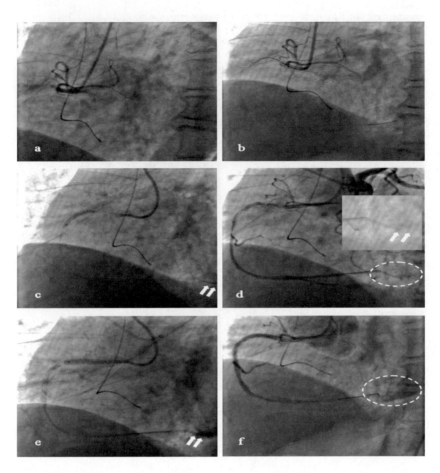

Figure 3-30 CAP caused by guidewire during PCI of right coronary occlusion. a: The proximal RCA was completely occluded; b: Crosswire NT with parallel guidewire technology passes through the occluded lesion to the distal RCA; c: Ryujin balloon (2.5 mm × 20 mm) expand the lesion of RCA. At this time, the head of the guidewire is located at the distal RCA (arrow); d: The operator immediately withdrew the guidewire, but there was a small amount of myocardial staining (see the arrow in the local enlarged image); e: Myocardial staining gradually increased, but at this time, the patient's hemodynamics was stable. Immediate Echo on bedside showed that there was a small amount of pericardial effusion, and there was no pressure on RV, so interventional therapy was continued; f: After the operation, the myocardial staining did not expand further, and the patient's Bp was stable. Echo was followed-up for 3 times after the operation, and there was no pressure on RV and no increase in pericardial effusion.

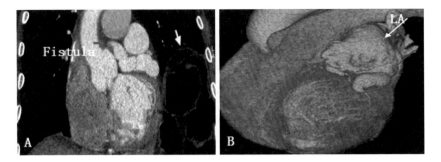

Figure 3-31 A: Course of the CAF (red arrow). A huge diaphragmatic hernia is also shown (white arrow); B: Markedly dilated LM and tortuous proximal portion of the first diagonal artery (red arrow).

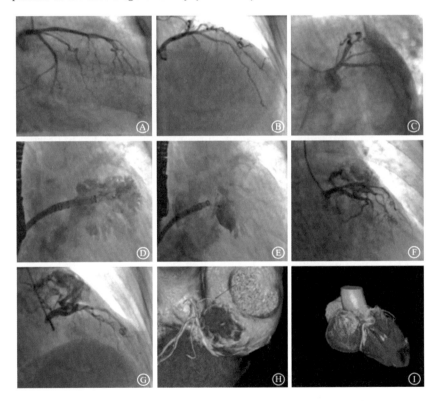

Figure 3-32 A & C: ICA showed normal LCX; D & E: LAA occlusion; F & G: In post-operation, LCX-LAA fistula was found; H & I: CTA showed 2 small branches from LCX to LAA. And normal occluder shadow can be seen in LAA.

Chapter IV   Pathology

Highlights

- The pathological anatomy of congenital CAF is characterized by abnormal communication between the coronary artery with non-capillary bed and the cardiac cavity, CS or its branches, SVC, PA, and pulmonary vein.
- The heart of CAF patient can expand to varying degrees. LV is often dilated and thickened, and sometimes RV is also thickened. The proximal coronary artery is tortuous and dilated, and the origin of abnormal coronary artery is enlarged, but the terminal fistula is usually small.
- The most common CAF is from RCA and LAD, while LCX fistula is rare. The most common drainage site is RV, RA, or PA, and it rarely terminates in the left side of the heart, but when it does, LA is the first.
- Most of them are isolated but often associated with other CAA (25%), such as pulmonary or aortic atresia, PDA, and VSD.
- The location of CAF: RCA fistula, LCA fistula, bilateral CAF, and single CAF; Drainage site of CAF: RV, RA (including CS and SVC), PA, LA, and LV.
- The coronary artery with abnormal communication is significantly dilated and distorted, and its wall is as thin as vein, which can form AN, and thrombus can form in AN.

CAF are congenital or acquired communications between the coronary arteries and, most commonly, RV, RA, or PA, although they can communicate with other cardiac structures. The majority of these defects are minor and hemodynamically insignificant. CHF may occur early in the infant if the fistula is large and results in volume overload and pulmonary hypertension. In large shunts, there may also be coronary steal phenomenon and myocardial ischemia. The involved coronary artery can dilate significantly to compensate for the shunt volume, but this can ultimately increase the risk of AN, rupture, ulceration, branch occlusion, atheroma, and calcification of the vessel. If untreated, large CAF can result in chronic myocardial ischemia, angina, cardiomyopathy, CHF, AMI, arrhythmia, and endocarditis (Figure 4-1).

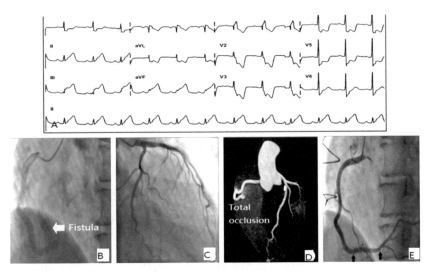

Figure 4-1   A: ECG showed ST segment elevation in lead Ⅱ, Ⅲ, and aVF; B: The RCA fistula; C: Normal LCA; D: Total occlusion of RCA; E: Normal RCA after operation.

1. Pathology of CAF

In 1908, Abbott M first described the pathological changes of CAF, which can occur in one of the 3 main coronary arteries and any segment and can involve LM. Many doctors in China reported some complex and rare cases (Figures 4-2, 4-3, and 4-4), such as Han D, Shen A, Xiang H, and Yu L. Some domestic scholars summarized the involved coronary artery of nearly 300 cases of CAF, 55% were involved in RCA and its branches, 35% in LCA, and 5% in both.

About 90% of CAF flows into the venous system, and more than 90% of cases have left-right shunt. The low-pressure area of the cardiac cavity is the common drainage site of CAF, such as the right cardiac cavity, PA, SVC,

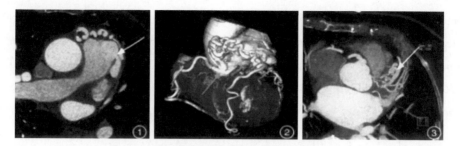

Figure 4-2　CT images of bilateral CAF. ① The PA fistula (arrow); ② The RCA is abnormally dilated and tortuous (arrow); ③ The oblique cross-sectional reconstruction image showed that the abnormal branch is connected with LAD (arrow).

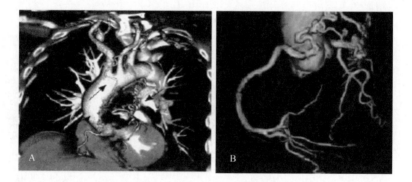

Figure 4-3　A: CT image of RCA and left internal mammary artery-PA fistula; B: CT finding of double CAPF.

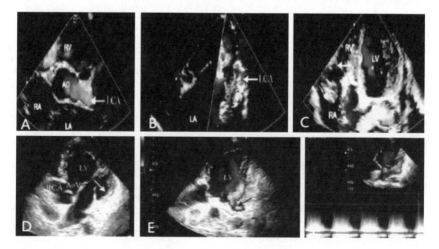

Figure 4-4　A-C: Echo of LCA-RV fistula; D-F: Echo of RCA-LV fistula.

and CS (Figure 4-5). Fistula communicating with the left cardiac cavity is rare. Foreign scholars reported that 41% of CAF drained into RV, 26% of RA, 17% of PA, 3% of LV and 1% of SVC (Figures 4-6, 4-7, and 4-8). Farand P reported a case of bridging vessel-CS fistula after CABG (Figure 4-9).

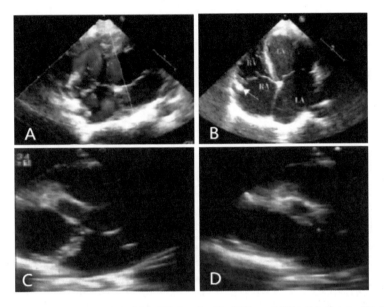

Figure 4-5   Echo findings of RCA-RV fistula (A & B) and RCA-RA fistula (C & D).

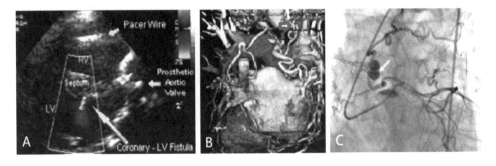

Figure 4-6   A: Echo of coronary artery-LV fistula (yellow arrow); B & C: CT image (red arrow) and angiogram (white arrow) of LCX-bronchial artery fistula.

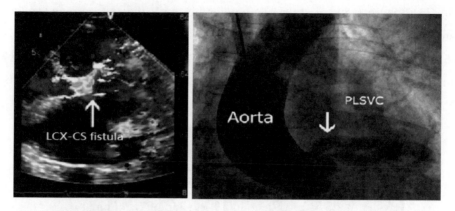

Figure 4-7   Echo and angiogram of LCX-CS fistula with persistent left superior vena cava (PLSVC).

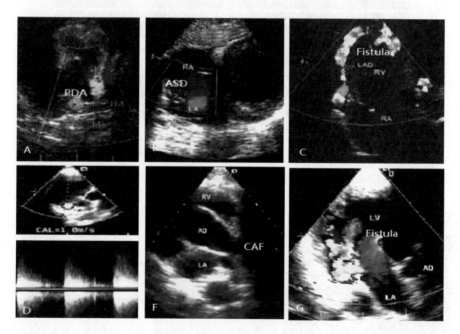

Figure 4-8   A-C: Echo of PDA, ASD and LCA-RV fistula; D-F: Echo of LCA-LV fistula.

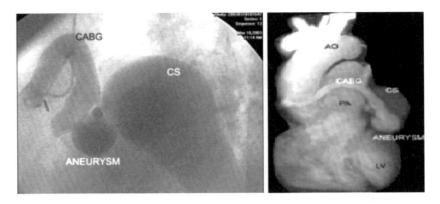

Figure 4-9   Angiography and MRI examination of bridging vessel-CS fistula after CABG.

Some scholars have summarized the characteristics of CCF: RCA fistula often runs along the right atrioventricular junction, and LCA fistula often runs along the left atrioventricular junction. The section of the fistula can be seen locally, and the involved vessel is often dilated and tortuous (Figures 4-10, 4-11).

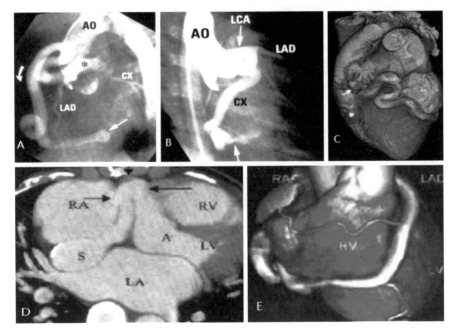

Figure 4-10   Angiogram and CT images of CCF. A-C: RCA-RV fistula; D: RCA-RA fistula; E: LAD-RV/RA fistula.

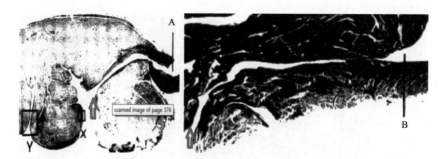

Figure 4-11　Pathological changes of CCF. A & B: The origin of CCF; Red arrows are outlet of CCF.

Shi Z reported 2 cases of prenatally diagnosed isolated CAF (Figures 4-12, 4-13). The first fetus had a fistulous communication between LCX and RA, and the second fetus had RCA-LV fistula.

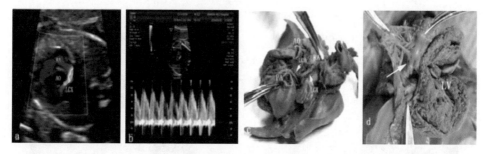

Figure 4-12　CDFI showed CAF draining into RA and originating from the dilated LCA a: Red represents blood flow toward Echo probe and blue means blood flow away the probe); b: Pulsed Doppler revealed biphasic forward blood flow; c: Gross dissection demonstrated the enlarged, dominant LCX, draining into the top of RA; d: Showed the orifice of LCX in RA (arrow).

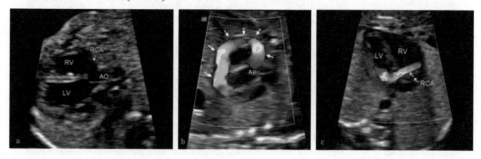

Figure 4-13　RCA was markedly dilated (a); CDFI showed the course of RCA (white arrow in b); CDFI showed the drainage of RCA in LV (c).

Acquired CAF or CAP are mostly secondary to surgery, such as left-left shunt after surgery of the outflow tract in hypertrophic obstructive cardiomyopathy (HOCM). Chenzbraun A retrospectively analyzed the Echo examination of 26 patients with HOCM after septal myectomy. The results showed that the incidence of CAF was 19%. The probability of CAF after septal myectomy was much higher than predicted and easily missed. Liang S, Konings TC, and Lee C reported several cases of CAF after PCI, TOF surgery, and endocardial biopsy (Figures 4-14, 4-15 and 4-16).

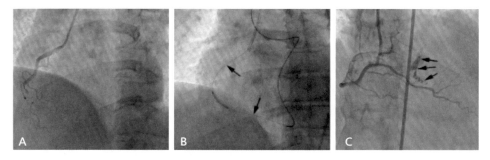

Figure 4-14   A: The CTO of RCA; B: After successful retrograde wire crossing, externalization was achieved with guidewire (arrow); C: RCA revealed Ellis type Ⅲ septal collateral perforation (arrows) into RV.

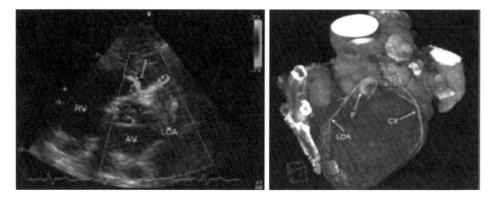

Figure 4-15   Echo and CT image of LCA-RV fistula after TOF surgery

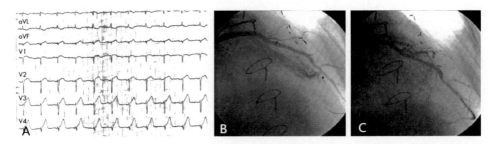

Figure 4-16 CAF and AMI after endocardial biopsy. A: ECG showed AMI; B: Angiographic changes of LCA fistula; C: Angiography after covered stent implantation.

Shriti M reported one case with orbital atherectomy-induced CAF (Figure 4-17). Saeko Y described an autopsy case of multiple coronary artery microfistulas (CAMF) in a 16-year-old girl, which was detected by ICA 5 years after she underwent Fontan surgery (the first choice of surgery in the treatment of patients with functional single ventricle). The autopsied heart revealed multiple dilated vessels with unique shape within the ventricular myocardium. Pathological features were consistent with those of residual sinusoidal, thereby causing CAMF (Figure 4-18).

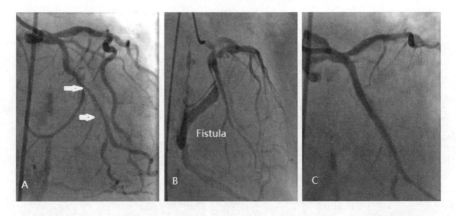

Figure 4-17 A: ICA revealed a calcified 90% proximal to mid LCX stenosis; B: ICA revealed patent LCX stents and a fistula between proximal/mid LCX and CS/venous system; C: The fistula was successfully excluded with the placement of 2 covered stents.

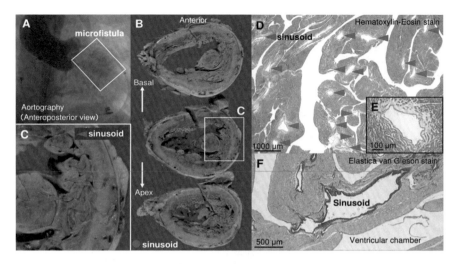

Figure 4-18　Aortogram and pathological findings. A: Aortogram showed CAMF (white box); B: Mapping of CAMF (red circle) in gross images of autopsied heart; C: Enlarged Figure B, with arrowheads indicated CAMF; D-F: Histological images of CAMF stained with hematoxylin-eosin (D & E) and Elastica van Gieson (F).

2. Pathology of AN

Coronary artery dilatation is very common in patients with CAF, and the degree of dilatation is not always consistent with the shunt flow (Figure 4-19). When the shunt occurs at the distal end of the coronary artery, the diameter of the artery may not change significantly. Most cases are single fistula, and multiple fistulas have also been reported (Figure 4-20). When coronary fistula drains into PA, the shunt flow is usually small.

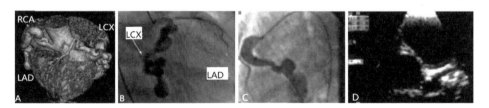

Figure 4-19　A & B: CT image and angiogram of LCX and RCA-RA fistula; C & D: Angiogram and Echo of CAF with AN.

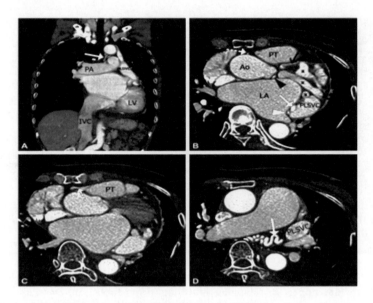

Figure 4-20 CT images of multiple CAF. A: PLSVC and descending aorta-left bronchial artery fistula; B: LAD, LCX and sinus node branch-bronchial artery fistula, RCA-PA fistula; C: RCA-PA fistula; D: Descending aorta-left bronchial artery fistula, and PLSVC.

The most common cause of AN is atherosclerosis, and non-atherosclerotic causes of giant AN include connective tissue disorder, vasculitis, infection, drug abuse, and trauma. However, the precise mechanism of giant AN associated with CAF is unknown. Until 2022, more than 15 previous case reports of histological changes of giant AN (defined as diameter ≥ 2 cm) associated with CAF. The histological changes were as followings: atherosclerosis, mucoid degeneration with infiltration of inflammatory cells, both atherosclerosis and mucoid degeneration, dysplastic medial change, and degenerative change with fatty infiltration and calcification. There was no difference in the incidence of histological changes among different coronary arteries or fistula-draining sites.

Sakata N suggested that a structural change of CAF, such as disrupted internal elastic lamina and phenotypic changes of the medial smooth muscle cells, might contribute to the aneurysmal formation (7-8 mm in diameter). Thus, wall weakness related to medial degeneration, in addition to insufficiency of internal and /or external elastic lamina of the CAF may have contributed to the development of the giant AN.

In conclusion, the structural abnormality of the fistula wall unrelated to atherosclerosis and mucoid degeneration may be one of the mechanisms underlying giant aneurysmal formation in patients with CAF.

Matsumoto Y presented a case of giant AN, LCA-PA fistula with deficiency of internal and /or external elastic lamina and medial degeneration (Figures 4-21, 4-22).

Studies have shown that these abnormal coronary arteries with malformations have thick intima and tight arrangement of smooth muscle cells. Abnormal arterial α-Smooth muscle actin (SMA), Calmodulin, and Desmin staining were positive, and endothelial cells were CD34 positive. Usually, abnormalities are accompanied by AN dilatation in the neck of the abnormal coronary artery.

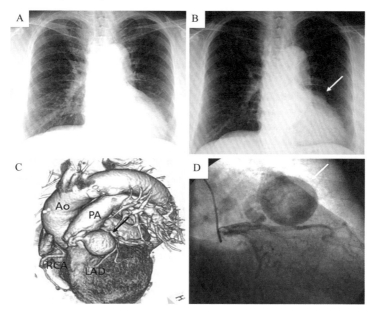

Figure 4-21   Chest X-ray showed a bulge in the third arch of the left heart border (B, arrow), although there was no observable mass on the chest X-ray taken 7 years ago (A); CTA (C) and angiogram (D) showed the giant AN (3 cm in diameter) (arrow) and LAD-PA fistula.

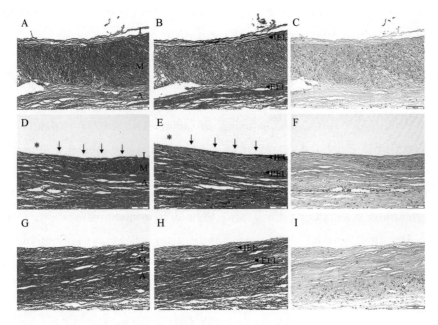

Figure 4-22 In the fistula conduit from LAD, the wall consisted of almost normal arterial structure containing intima (I), internal elastic lamina (IEL), media (M), external elastic lamina (EEL), and adventitia (A) with mild intimal thickening (A & B) and mild degeneration and deposition of Alcian blue-positive materials in the media (C). However, the wall of AN had a gradual decrease of smooth muscle cells in the media (D & E, arrows) with a lack of EEL from the entry of the fistula conduit from the LAD to the distal site (E, arrowhead of EEL), and about 15mm from the entry of the fistula conduit from LAD (D&E, asterisk), the media and IEL disappeared and changed to fibrosis without inflammatory cells (D & E). Moreover, the remaining of the aneurysmal wall had been almost completely transformed by fibrosis, in addition to disrupted EEL with preserved internal elastic lamina (IEL) (G & H). Deposition of Alcian blue-positive materials was also seen in the aneurysmal wall (F-I).

Due to the formation of AN, in the diastolic period of the heart, blood is deposited in AN, which can compress the myocardium and distal coronary artery and cause myocardial ischemia. Thrombosis can also occur in AN, and distal coronary embolism or AMI can be caused by thrombus, especially in the patients with atrial fibrillation. The heart of patients with congenital CAF can expand to varying degrees, especially LV swells and thickens, and the ascending aorta also magnifies. On the surface of the heart, the involved coronary artery dilates and twists, and the vessel wall becomes thinner, sometimes forming spindle AN. Milici C and Katayama T reported 2 cases with CAF and giant AN (Figures 4-23, 4-24), and Sakata N reported the

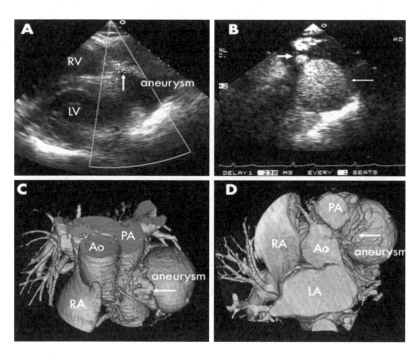

Figure 4-23   Echo and CT image of LAD fistula with giant AN.

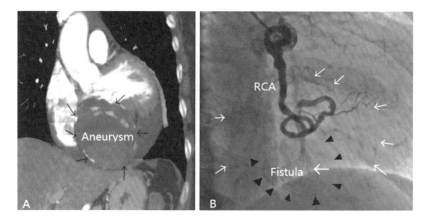

Figure 4-24   CT image and angiogram of RCA fistula with aneurysmal dilatation.

histopathological characteristics of LCA-PA fistula with aneurysmal dilatation (Figures 4-25, 4-26).

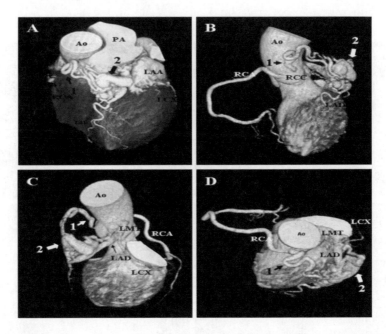

Figure 4-25 CT image of LCA-PA fistula with aneurysmal dilatation.
1: Fistula; 2: AN.

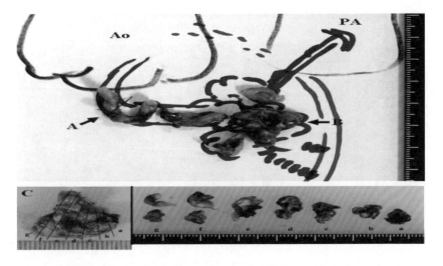

Figure 4-26 Pathological changes of LCA-PA fistula with AN.

RCA-LV fistula with giant AN is an extremely rare cardiac condition. Diao W presents a patient with large LV and giant AN with a maximal inner diameter of approximately 56.6 mm and 22 mm. The patient underwent surgical management by suturing of proximal end of AN and CABG (Figures 4-27, 4-28).

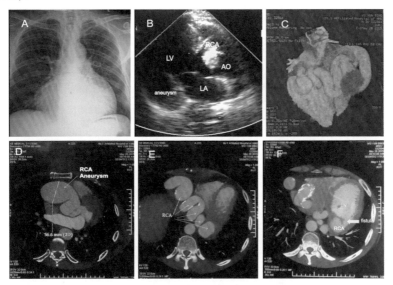

Figure 4-27　A: Chest X-ray showed a significant expansion on the right and left cardiac border; B: TTE revealed a huge RCA aneurysm; C: CT showed AN; D-F: CT scan showed RCA being wholly dilated and a fistula at LV.

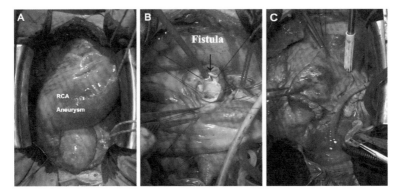

Figure 4-28　A: Aneurysmal sac and RCA; B: RCA ostium was demonstrated by the arrow; C: Closure of the beginning of RCA ostium with a vein graft to the distal RCA.

RCA-LV fistula with giant AN may eventuate serious complications, such as thrombosis, rupture, and CHF. Therefore, it is necessary to establish effective management strategies for this condition. Although this case is not unique, it serves as an illustrative example of the implementation of a classic surgical treatment method.

Crawley PD believed that the incidence of giant AN (>20 mm) was 0.02%– 0.2% , and the common causes included atherosclerosis, Takayasu arteritis, Kawasaki disease, complications of PCI, and congenital factors. Pallisgaard JL reported a 62-year-old female patient with chest pain. CT and angiogram showed LAD-PA fistula with giant AN formation. Schmack B and Bernhardt AM also reported several cases of giant RCA/LCX-CS fistula with successful surgical treatment (Figure 4-29).

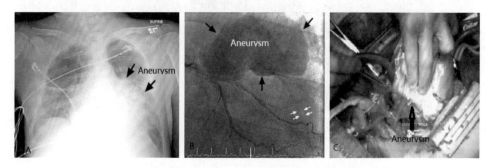

Figure 4-29 A & B: Chest X-ray and angiographic changes of giant AN; C: Operative field of coronary artery-CS fistula.

Mori A reported an asymptomatic 75-year-old woman with a 40 mm, round-shaped lesion beside PA on CT. ICA showed LAD-PA fistula with AN. The aneurysm was resected with CABG successfully. Pathological analysis revealed that medial depletion similar to segmental arterial mediolysis (SAM) might contribute to aneurysm formation (Figure 4-30).

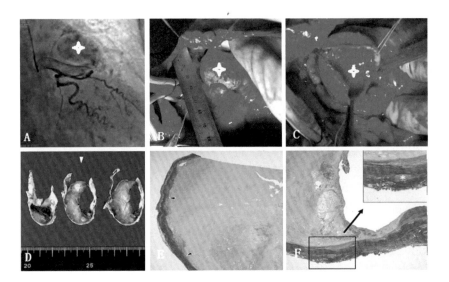

Figure 4-30   Pathological analysis after surgery of LAD-PA fistula with AN. A: ICA
showed LAD-PA fistula, dilated LM and AN; B & C: Intra-operative inspection of
calcified, egg-shaped mass between the base of PA and LCA; D: Macroscopic
findings. Cross-sections of resected AN showed uneven thickness of the arterial
wall, accompanied by calcification. The inside of AN is filled with thrombus. The
second slice from the left (white arrow) is explored using light microscopy;
E: Thinnest AN wall where the media is extensively defective (black arrows). The
inside of AN is filled with atherosclerotic thrombus; F: Most parts of AN consist of
adventitia and intima. The media is found (asterisk) segmentally.

Chapter V Pathophysiology

Highlights

- CAF makes the coronary blood flow directly shunt into the cardiac cavity or vessel, forming an invalid circulation, increasing the cardiac load, and reducing the distal coronary blood supply.

- The shunt volume depends on CAF size and drainage site into the cardiac cavity or vessel. If draining into the atrium, the shunt flow is large because the pressure in the atrium is low, the atrium wall is thin, and the fistula does not shrink with the contraction of the heart. If draining into the ventricle, the shunt flow is minor.

- Because LV pressure is higher than RV, the shunt flow into LV is smaller than that into RV. Once CAF branch flows into the right cardiac system, it will form a left-right shunt, which can cause pulmonary congestion and hypertension, LV and/or RV hypertrophy. If the branch flows into LV system, it will only cause LV overload and hypertrophy.

- CAF causes damage to the intima and pathological changes such as arteriosclerosis, AN, IE, and thrombosis. The dilated tortuous coronary artery can also easily form the mural thrombus, rupture, etc. These changes tend to worsen with the patient's age.

Left-right shunt of both systolic and diastolic phases was found in patients with CAF draining into the right heart system, which was similar to the pathophysiological changes of PDA and AN of aortic sinuses, such as pulmonary hypertension, LV dilatation, hypertrophy, and CHF (Figures 5-1, 5-2). However, fewer of them cause the pulmonary/systemic blood flow ratio (Qp/Qs) to be greater than 1.8. There was no left-right but left-left shunt in the patients with CAF draining to the left heart system. In the patients with coronary artery-LV fistula, there was a shunt only in the

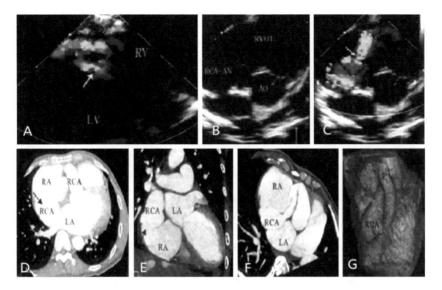

Figure 5-1   RCA fistula with tumor-like dilatation. A-C: The proximal apical segment of RCA was enlarged in tumor-like manner. The arrow showed the site of the fistula, which was located within AN; D-G: CT scan of RCA-RA fistula with AN.

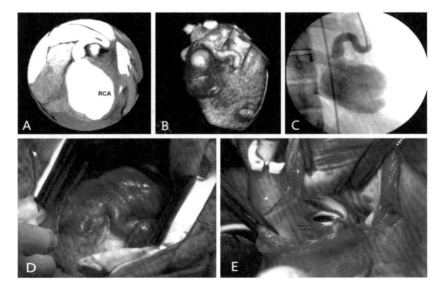

Figure 5-2   CT images (A & B), angiogram (C) and surgical field of giant AN with RCA-RV fistula (D & E).

diastolic phase, but there was a continuous (systolic and diastolic phase) shunt in the patients with coronary artery-LA fistula. Both of the above can form pathophysiological changes similar to aortic regurgitation.

CAF includes abnormal communications between the coronary arteries and cardiac chambers, referred to as CCF, or abnormal communications between the coronary arteries and other vessels, referred to as CAVF. According to hemodynamics, there are also 2 main types (Figures 5-3, 5-4): coronary arteriovenous fistula (CAVF, communicating with the right heart system) and internal fistula of systemic circulation (CAF, communicating with the left heart system).

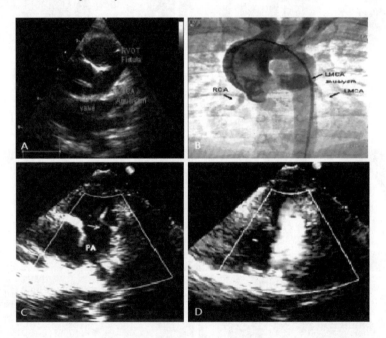

Figure 5-3 A & B: Echo and angiogram of LM-RV fistula; C: Pre-operative LCA-PA fistula; D: No abnormal blood flow in PA after surgery.

A fistula originating from RCA draining into RV is the most common type of CAF. Most fistula terminate into RV or RA. Rarely do they terminate into LA or LV. Congenital or acquired CCF are infrequent anomalies with a wide spectrum of clinical presentation that may vary from asymptomatic to severely devastating states requiring different treatment modalities. The

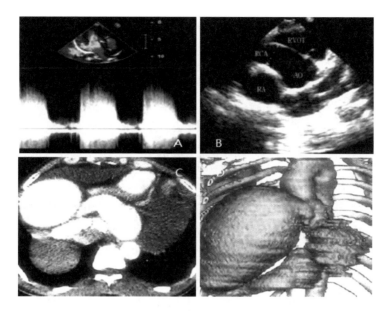

Figure 5-4   The RCA-LV fistula. A & B: Echo showed the dilated RCA; C & D: The giant tumor-like dilatation of RCA was tortuous, descending along the right margin of the heart, communicating with LV via the posterior wall, and pericardial effusion was seen.

treatment choice depends on whether CCF is congenital or acquired. Whereas congenital CAMF can be treated medically with β-blocker or calcium channel blocker, a large solitary fistula that leads to severe hemodynamic shunts should be closed by transcatheter or surgical means.

Patients with CAF can present with myocardial ischemia or coronary steal phenomenon, which is explained by a pressure gradient between the diastolic coronary artery and the fistula outlet connecting the cardiac cavity or vessel. If the fistula is large, the diastolic pressure of this coronary artery can be progressively reduced by exercise, because of obviously increased oxygen demand, distal myocardial ischemia, and hypoxia. Therefore, the nutrient artery from the sinus ostium to CAF will become severe with age, leading to calcification, thrombosis, and even rupture (Figure 5-5).

Hemodynamic changes depend on the size of the fistula, the location of the fistula, the resistance of the abnormal coronary artery, the pressure

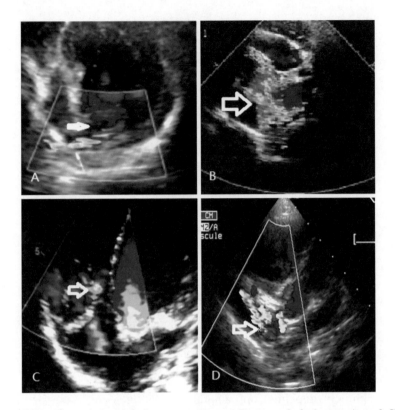

Figure 5-5 The relationship between shunt volume and drainage site of CAF
A: RCA-LV fistula; B: RCA-LA fistula; C: RCA-RV fistula; D: RCA-RA fistula.

gradient between the cardiac cavity and blood vessel, and whether there are other malformations. At first, the pathophysiological changes of CAF depend on the resistance between the coronary artery and the site where the fistula drains. The resistance is due to the fastula's length, size, and tortuosity.

The types of CAF entering the cardiac cavity or vein:

a. CAF is generally single fistula;

b. Multiple fistula orifices or vascular plexus;

c. The fistula is located on the side of the main branch and forms a communication with the cardiac cavity, or the coronary artery expands significantly, forming AN. The exact location and size of CAF cannot be determined from the surface of the heart.

CAF results in a left-right (over 90%) or left-left shunt (Table 5-1). A small fistula is not of hemodynamic significance. However, larger fistulae can lead to hemodynamic compromise by the coronary steal phenomenon, which occurs from decreased myocardial blood flow. With a large fistula, the diastolic perfusion pressure inside the coronary vessel progressively decreased. The hemodynamic consequences of the shunt are related to the amount of blood flow from the fistula to the chamber and the resistance of the fistula blood flow.

Table 5-1   Hemodynamic consequences and complications for each shunt type

Shunt type	Hemodynamic consequences		Complications
Left-right (coronary artery to right vessels/ chambers)	Continuous flow for all cardiac cycle durations due to lower pressure in the right structure (vessel or chamber) compared to the smaller arterioles and capillaries of the myocardium.	Coronary steal phenomenon due to blood diastolic run-off directed away from the normal coronary circulation and myocardial microcirculation.	Volume overload of both ventricles or, generally, cardiac chambers.
Left-left (LA or pulmonary vein)	Continuous flow for all the cardiac cycle due to lower pressure in LA/pulmonary vein compared to the smaller arterioles and capillaries of the myocardium.		Volume overload of left chambers only.
Left-left (LV)	Blood run-off from the aorta.		Volume overload of left chambers mimicking the mechanisms of aortic valve regurgitation.

When a fistula drains to the right side of the circulation, there is usually a ting-to-moderate shunt. For instance, those that drain to RA will have physiological changes similar to ASD, and those that drain to PA will have physiological changes similar to PDA. When the fistula drains into LA, the physiology would be volume load similar to mitral regurgitation, and also similar to aortic regurgitation with drainage into LV (Figure 5-6).

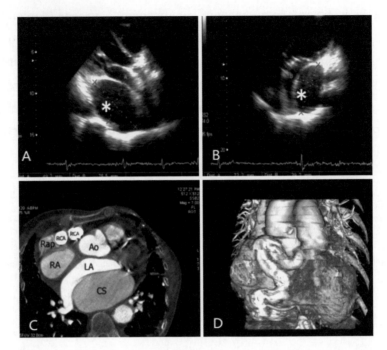

Figure 5-6　Echo (A & B) and CT images (C & D) of RCA-CS fistula.
＊ The size of AN was 49.2 mm × 78.5 mm.

When the blood flow of CAF drains into a left-side chamber, it produces blood run-off from the aorta simulating aortic regurgitation followed by volume overload that, over time, could lead to dilatation of the heart chambers. The clinical consequences of the volume overload may be CHF, atrial and ventricular tachyarrhythmia. Very rarely, mainly in adults, ischemia occurs in the myocardial territory beyond the fistula's origin due to increased myocardial oxygen demand, and this usually presents with symptoms during physical activity (Figure 5-7).

CAF can be large and dilated or ectatic, up to 250 mm in diameter, and these tend to become wider over time. A persistent high-speed flow in coronary arteries may cause massive dilatation and AN formation. Premature coronary atherosclerosis is also reported. Valvular regurgitation due to papillary muscle dysfunction is possible in children and adults with CAF. Hemopericardium can occur due to the rupture of AN. Very rarely,

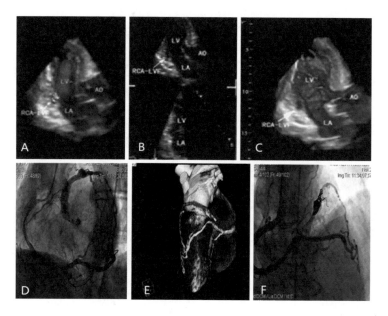

Figure 5-7　A-C: Echo of RCA-LV fistula; D-F: Comparison before and after TCC with detachable coil.

pulmonary hypertension may result in a left-right shunt. Symptoms and sequela include chronic myocardial ischemia, angina, AMI and CHF.

CHF is the consequence of long-term persistent massive shunt. After the age of 40, about 3/4 of patients have different degrees of symptoms. It is important to note that CHF occurs in patients who communicate with RV. Although the left-right shunt of a large fistula can cause mild-to-moderate pulmonary hypertension, no Eisenmenger syndrome has been reported.

Lee WS reported a bronchiectasis patient who presented with hemoptysis and AMI was confirmed by CT and angiography as having RCA-bronchial artery fistula. Kurt IH reported a case of AMI due to LAD-LV fistula (Figures 5-8, 5-9).

Different drainage sites can cause different cardiac loads. If communicating with PA only caused LV overload; communicating with RV, the volume load of the chamber tended to increase; communicating directly with RA, the volume load of both RA and RV changed. Whether draining to RA or RV, the shunting blood needs to pass through the pulmonary vascular

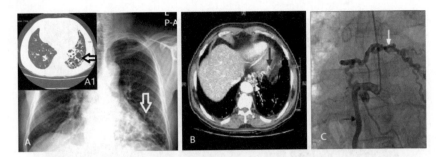

Figure 5-8 A & A1: Chest X-ray and CT images of the bronchiectasis (left lower lung field, white and black arrow); B & C: RCA-bronchial artery fistula.

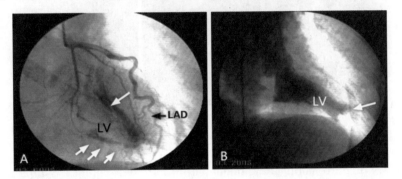

Figure 5-9 Coronary angiogram (A) and left ventriculogram (B) of LAD-LV fistula.

bed before reaching the coronary artery and then into LA and LV, so it must also increase the volume load of the left heart system (Figures 5-10, 5-11).

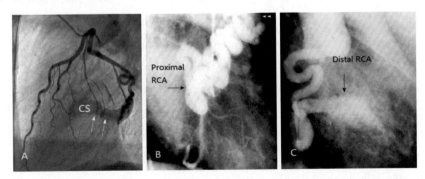

Figure 5-10 A: Angiographic changes of LCX-CS fistula; B: Proximal RCA-PA fistula with dilated coronary artery; C: Distal RCA-LV fistula with dilated coronary artery.

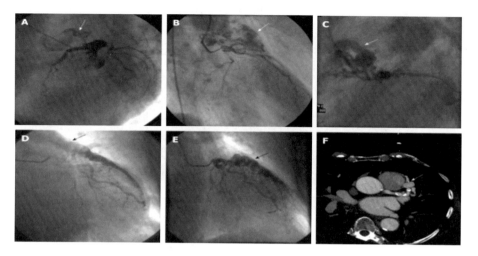

Figure 5-11   Various types of LCA-PA fistula. A: Single origin and ostium, tortuous fistula; B: Multiple origins and ostia; C: Multiple origin and ostia, with aneurysmal dilatation; D & E: Dilated and tortuous LAD-PA fistula; F: CT showed LAD-PA fistula.

Oylumlu M reported a case of myocardial ischemia due to 3 major CCF (Figure 5-12).   Co-existing   cardiovascular   malformations   aggravate hemodynamics and affect the patient's prognosis. Lee JJ reported a case of TOF with CAF (Figure 5-13).

Zhang G and Chang H analyzed the clinical symptoms, ECG, Echo findings, and coronary angiographic characteristics of patients with CAMF (Figure 5-14). From 1998 to 2008, coronary artery-LV microvascular fistulas were found in 9 patients (mean age 71.5 years), and 7 of them (77.8%) were female. All patients were admitted because of angina-like chest tightness and shortness of breath. CAD was found in 5 cases (55.6%), hypertension in 2 cases (22.2%), valvular heart disease and cardiomyopathy in 1 case (11.1%) each, respectively. Microvascular fistula originated from one coronary artery in 1 case (11.1%), 2 coronary arteries in 6 cases (66.7%), and 3 coronary arteries in 2 cases (22.2%). All patients had fistulas originating from the diagonal branch. On ICA, the contrast media diffused directly to LV via microvascular fistula and showed the image of cardiac cavity staining. The authors believe that CAMF is more common in women, and microvascular

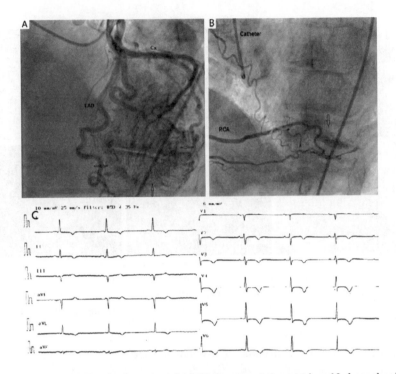

Figure 5-12 A & B: Angiogram of multiple coronary arteries (3 branches)-LV fistula; C: ECG showed ischemic T wave invevion in the anterior wall.

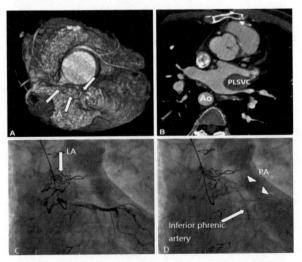

Figure 5-13 CT findings of TOF with CAF. A: LCA-LA fistula; B: PLSVC with dilated CS; C: LCA-LA fistula; D: LAD-inferior phrenic artery, collateral artery-PA communication.

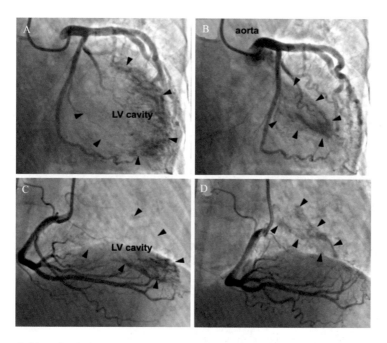

Figure 5-14   Angiogram showed normal epicardial vessels, and the sequence demonstrated multiple fine fistulas draining to LV. As a result, a striking pattern of filling and emptying of this chamber is visualized during diastole (A & C) and systole (B & D), respectively (arrowheads indicate LV cavity). The fistula emerged from the proximal, mid, and distal segments of LAD and LCX (A).

fistula originating from 2 branches of coronary artery is the most common. And all patients with CAMF have fistulas originating from the diagonal branch.

Luis E reported a case with giant RCA aneurysm pouring into SVC. A 78-year-old woman was referred to the hospital with exertional chest pain, progressive dyspnea, and heart murmur. Her medical record was relevant with hypertension, dyslipidemia, and persistent atrial fibrillation. Physical examination revealed a loud continuous murmur at the left sternal border. On TTE, unusual flow originating from the right sinus of Valsalva was noted and confirmed with TEE. However, this artery was filled from LCA. Aortography revealed a giant para-aortic aneurysm. Oximetry showed increased oxygen saturation at the lower end of SVC, and the Qp/Qs ratio was calculated at

3.5:1. CT scan with 3D volume-rendering reconstruction showed a giant AN (7 cm in diameter) arising from the proximal segment of RCA, and injecting to SVC. Surgical intervention successfully resected AN and closed the fistula (Figure 5-15).

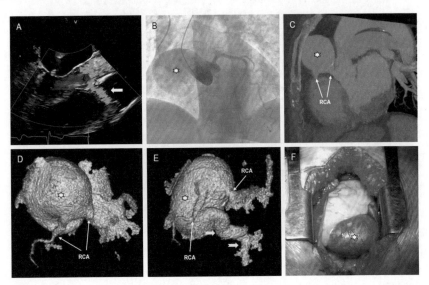

Figure 5-15   A: TEE showed turbulent flow originating from the right sinus of Valsalva (arrow); B: Aortography showed giant para-aortic aneurysm (star); C: CT scan showed giant AN (star) arising from the proximal RCA; D-E: CT scan showed the giant AN (star) arising from RCA, and the large fistula to SVC (notched arrows); F: Surgical exposure of AN (star).

An X presented a case with rare and complex CAPF, giant coronary aneurysmal dilatation, and thrombosis through multi-modality evaluations (Figure 5-16).

Campos ID presented the case of a 74-year-old woman with a previous history of hypercholesterolemia, hypertension, and atypical chest discomfort, who was admitted to the emergency department with severe retrosternal pain radiating to the left shoulder and dyspnea 2 hours after onset. On admission, physical examination was normal, with no signs of cardiac failure (Figure 5-17). The ECG showed a sinus rhythm with no pathological Q wave, abnormal ST segment, or T wave changes. Lab tests showed elevated cardiac

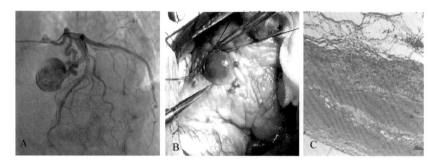

Figure 5-16　A: Coronary angiogram identified CAPF with giant aneurysmal dilation; B: AN with 3 cm in diameter located within the epicardial adipose tissue during surgery; C: Tissue biopsy of the coronary aneurysmal wall by Hematoxylin-Eosin staining showed moderate intimal fibrosis, degenerated media, and decreased smooth muscle layer.

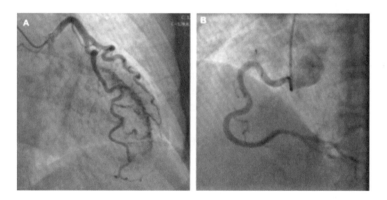

Figure 5-17　A: ICA showed multiple microfistulas from LCA to LV with no significant atherosclerotic stenosis; B: Normal RCA.

biomarkers (13ng/mL for troponin and 42IU/L for CK-MB).

Torres C described a case of bilateral coronary-PA fistula resulting in coronary steal syndrome after valve-sparing aortic repair surgery (Figure 5-18).

Erdogan E described a complex CAF leading to a myocardial steal. An Amplatzer occluder (vascular plug) via a transcatheter approach was utilized in managing this patient successfully without any complications (Figure 5-19).

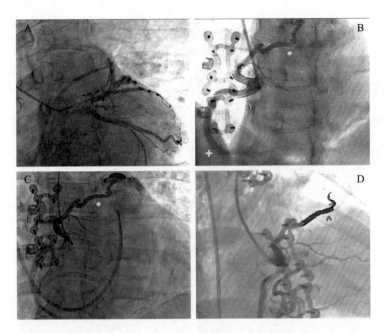

Figure 5-18 A: The yellow arrow demonstrated multiple small to moderatesized collateral originating proximally from LAD and anastomosing to the main PA; B & C: Demonstrated the true RCA (The large anomalous artery originating from RCA and anteriorly anastomosing to the main PA distally); D: Deployment (ˆ) of 2 Penumbra Ruby coils (3 mm × 20 cm and 3 mm × 15 cm) with no residual flow distally.

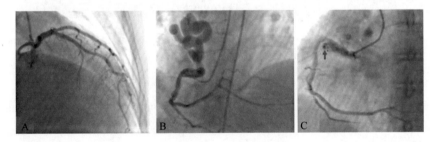

Figure 5-19 A: ICA showed normal LCA; B: Showed a giant tortuous CAF originating from the sinoatrial branch of RCA; C: Post-operative ICA showed almost completely occluded fistula. Vascular plug is seen in the ostium of fistula (red arrow).

Chapter VI   Classification and type

Highlights

• According to the origin, CAF is divided into right or left, single or multiple, and unspecified CAF.

• According to the drainage site, CAF is divided into coronary artery-RA or CS fistula, coronary artery-RV or PA fistula, and coronary artery-LA or LV fistula.

• Congenital CAF from RCA accounts for 50%–60%, from LCA accounts for 30%–40%, and from 2 coronary arteries for 2%–10%.

• The drainage site in the right cardiac system (RA, RV, PA, SVC, and coronary vein) accounts for 90%, in the left cardiac system (LA, LV) accounts for 10%, of which PA and RV is the most and LV is the least.

• There are 3 types of CAF entering the heart: single fistula; more than 2 fistulas; the fistula originating from LM to the cardiac cavity, or the coronary artery is obviously expanded to form AN.

At present, the classification of CAF has yet to be unified. Clinically, most of them are divided according to the origin of the coronary artery and the drainage site.

CAF can be divided into 2 categories:

—congenital (primary, hereditary);

—acquired (secondary, iatrogenic).

Lee SY reported a case of a giant RCA-CS fistula with PLSVC (Figure 6-1). Choi YJ reported an iatrogenic (acquired) CAF after ventricular septectomy of HOCM, which closed spontaneously after 3 months (Figure 6-2).

The CAF is a connection between one or more coronary arteries and cardiac chamber (CCF) or major blood vessel (CAVF) when the myocardial

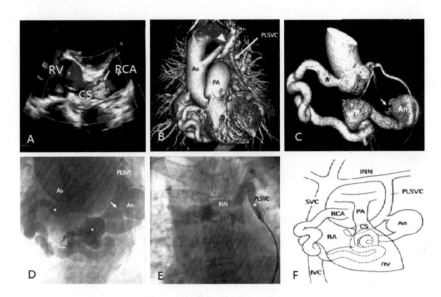

Figure 6-1　Congenital giant RCA-CS fistula with PLSVC. A: Echo showed RCA-CS fistula; B & C: CT images showed PLSVC and RCA-CS fistula with AN; D & E: Angiogram showed PLSVC and RCA-CS fistula with AN; F: Sketch map according to D angiogram.

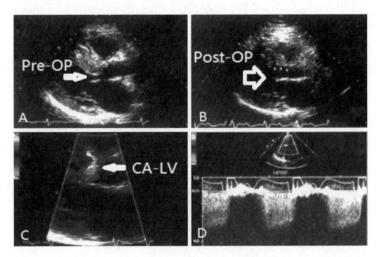

Figure 6-2　A: Ventricular septal hypertrophy with LVOT stenosis pre-operation; B: Hypertrophy and stenosis were reduced post-operation; C & D: Coronary artery-LV fistula post-operation.

capillary bed is bypassed. CAF is unilateral in most cases (more than 80%, both in children and adults), seldom bilateral or multilateral in very few cases.

Generally isolated (80%), they may also be associated with other CAA (20% , from 5% to 30%), including TOF, PDA, ASD and VSD. Said SAM. , Angelini P, Friedman AH and other scholars have conducted long-term researches on the type and classification of CAF and summarized the valuable experiences for clinical diagnosis and treatment (Figures 6-3, 6-4, 6-5, 6-6, and 6-7).

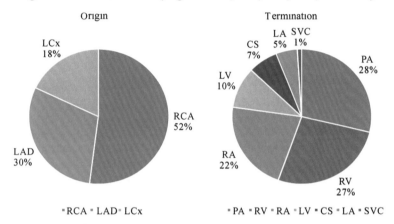

Figure 6-3   Common sites of origin and termination of CAF.

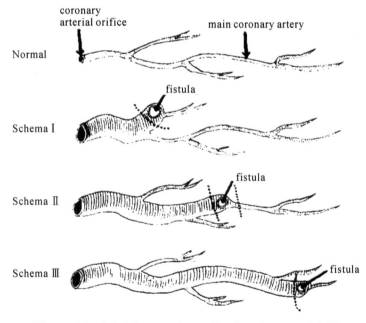

Figure 6-4   Sakakibara angiographic classification of CAF.

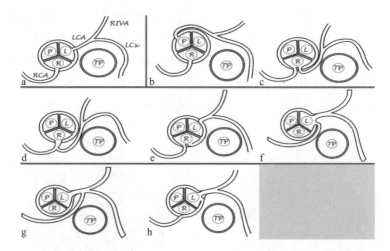

Figure 6-5   Various origins of CAA at coronary sinus. a: Normal anatomy; b: Anomalous origin of LCA from posterior sinus; c-h: ACAOS; c-e: Anomalous origin of LCA from RCS with interarterial course; c: Two ostia with separate origin of LCA and RCA from RCS; d: One ostium and common origin; e: Intramural course in the wall of aorta; f-h: Anomalous origin of RCA from LCS with interarterial course; Variants f-h comparable to c-e. ACAOS: the anomalous origin of coronary artery from the opposite sinus; LCS: left coronary sinus; RCS: right coronary sinus.

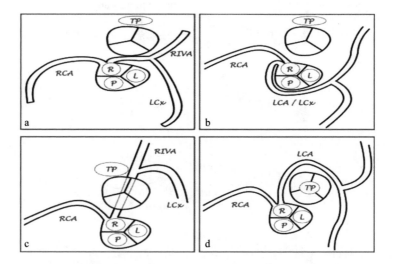

Figure 6-6   Variants of course in ACAOS (LCA from RCS). a: Interarterial course; b: Retroaortic course; c: Transseptal/sub-pulmonic course; d: Pre-pulmonic course.

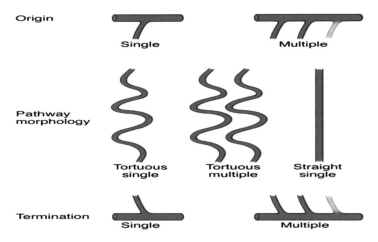

Figure 6-7   CAF anatomic classification system.

Fistulas commonly drain into the low-pressure right-side cardiac structure and less commonly drain into the left-side heart system. CAF with various drainage sites is illustrated in Figure 6-8.

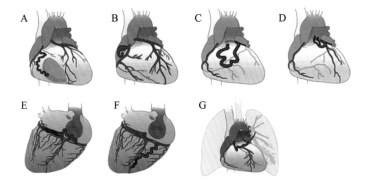

Figure 6-8   Classification of CAF based on the drainage site. A: CCF involving RV chamber; B: CCF involving RA chamber; C: CAPF involving single large fistulous tract; D: CAPF involving multiple small fistulous tracts; E: coronary artery-CS fistula; F: coronary artery-cardiac vein fistula; G: coronary artery-bronchial artery fistula.

Lee C retrospectively evaluated the demographics, clinical symptoms, and anatomical characteristics such as the origin, number of origins, course, opening site of the fistula, and the presence of aneurysmal changes (defined as dilatation 1.5 times of the origin). The authors also categorized the fistula openings according to the size compared to the proximal LAD. The patients were 14 men and 18 women with a mean (range) age of 56.5 (34-86) years. Nineteen patients had no related symptoms, and the others had symptoms such as angina, chest discomfort, palpitation, or shoulder pain. Among these patients, 2 patients were diagnosed with CAD. The origins of CAPF were single (n = 15, 46.9%) or multiple (n = 17, 53.1%). The CAPF arose most commonly from the conus branch of RCA (n = 20, 62.5%) and proximal LAD (n = 17, 53.1%). All fistulas coursed anteriorly to PA and drained into the anterolateral aspect. Twenty-five patients (78.1%) exhibited aneurysmal changes. The openings were small in 13 (40.6%), medium in 13 (40.6%), and large in 6 (18.8%) patients. More than half of patients with fistula had no related symptoms (Figures 6-9, 6-10, 6-11 and 6-12).

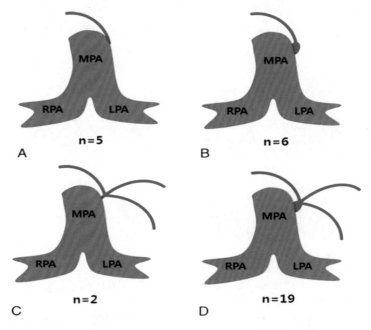

Figure 6-9 Schematic drawings of CAPF. A: Single origin without AN; B: Single origin with AN; C: Multiple origins without AN; D: Multiple origins with AN.

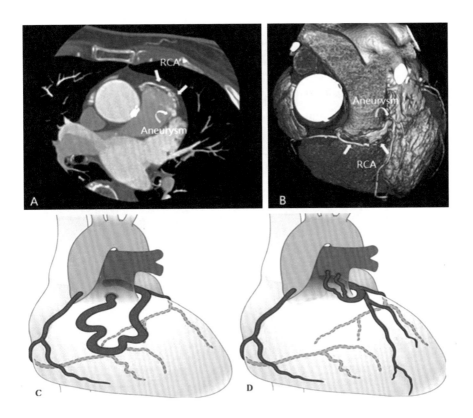

Figure 6-10   An 86-year-old woman without clinical symptoms who underwent CTA. CAPF originating from multiple origins of RCA (arrows) and the proximal LAD (not shown because of overlapping) was seen in both an axial image (A) and a 3-D reconstructed image (B). Combined AN was also noted (curved arrow). In (C) there was a single prominent fistulous connection between LM/LAD and PA, whereas in (D) there were multiple small-caliber fistulous connections between LM/LAD and PA. Although both types of CAPF involved the same vessels, anecdotally CAPF patients with morphology resembling (C) were more likely to be symptomatic as there was more significant hemodynamic effect when compared with CAPF patients with morphology resembling (D).

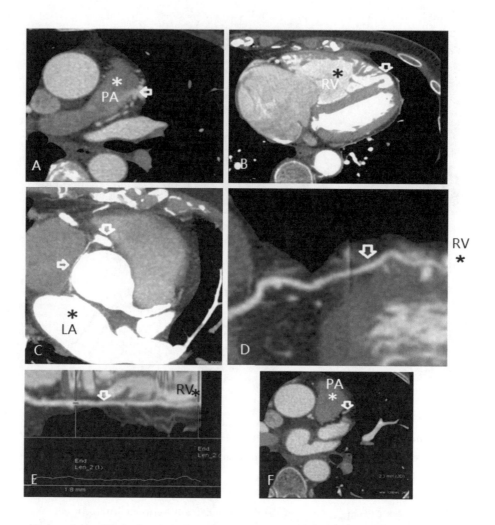

Figure 6-11 Methods of CAF evaluation; A: Mixed type fistula with aneurysmal widening and visible contrast jet to the PA (∗); B: Visible contrast intensity in RV apex, consistent with LCA fistula to RV (∗); C: Linear type fistula originating from RCA in maximum intensity projection (∗ LA); D: Example of LCA fistula to RV in curve reconstruction (∗ RV); E: Example of fistula's shortest distance of connection measurement in longitudinal reconstruction (∗ RV); F: Example of diameter measurement in LCA fistula (∗ PA).

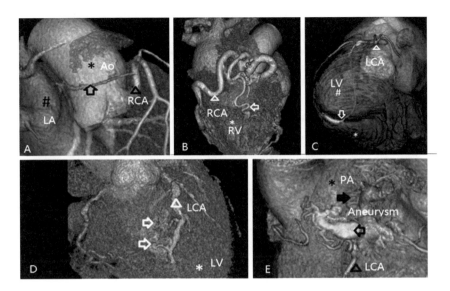

Figure 6-12　Types of CAF. A: Linear type fistula (arrow); B: Spiral type fistula (arrow); C: Aneurysmal type fistula (arrow); D: Grid-like type fistula (arrow); E: Mixed type fistula with AN.

Based on morphology, the simple CAF has a single origin and drains through one fistulous tract, whereas the complex CAF is composed of entangled blood vessels with multiple fistulous structures. Isolated CAF is found in 55%-80% of cases, whereas 5%-30% of cases involve other CAA. CAF classification according to various factors is listed in Figure 6-13 and Table 6-1.

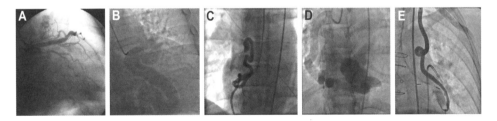

Figure 6-13　Types of CAF. A: Small LAD-PA fistula with weblike communications; B: Large distal LCX-CS fistula; C: Moderate-size RCA-SVC /RA fistula; D: Large RCA-CS fistula; E: Fistula from the left internal mammary artery (LIMA) to left PA.

Table 6-1   CAF classifications based on various factors

Classification	Description
Based on CAF etiology	Congenital: embryonic Acquired: —Iatrogenic: caused by PCI, CABG, cardiac transplantation, permanent pacemaker implantation, myocardial biopsy —Disease related: caused by AMI, cardiomyopathy (hypertrophic, dilated), Kawasaki disease, tumor —Trauma related: caused by penetrating or nonpenetrating trauma —Radiation injury
Based on CAF origin	RCA LCA: LAD and its branches, LCX and its branches, Ramus intermedius RCA and LCA Other anomalous coronary arteries
Based on segment of CAF origin	Sakakibara type A: originating from the proximal native vessel; distal artery is normal Sakakibara type B: originating from distal native vessel; the entire coronary artery is dilated
Based on drainage site	CCF: involving any cardiac chamber (RA, RV, LA, LV) CAVF: involving PA, CS, superior and inferior vena cava, bronchial vessel, other extracardiac veins (eg, azygos, costal, brachiocephalic veins)
Based on the number of fistulous tracts	Single or multiple
Based on CAF morphology and complexity	Simple CAF: has a single origin and drains through single vascular course Complex CAF: involves entangled blood vessels with multiple fistulous structures
Based on the presence of accompanying anomaly	Isolated CAF: no accompanying anomaly Combined CAF: accompanied by VSD, PDA, TOF, or other valvular disease

Tamer Y reported an extremely rare case of a 14-month-old girl diagnosed with single RCA-RV fistula and congenital absence of LCA. ICA showed a dilated and tortuous single RCA draining into RV, absence of left coronary system, and LV supplied via collateral vessels (Figure 6-14).

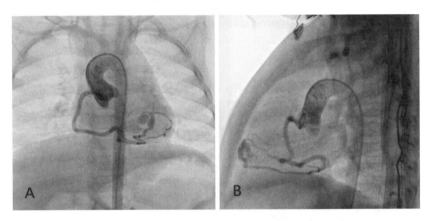

Figure 6-14   Aortic root injection. A: Dilated and tortuous vessel arises from the right CS, and LCA was undetected. There was a fistula leading to RV apex; B: Thin collateral vessels were supplying LCA territory.

Jan D reported a case with septal CAF following the left bundle branch area pacing (Figure 6-15).

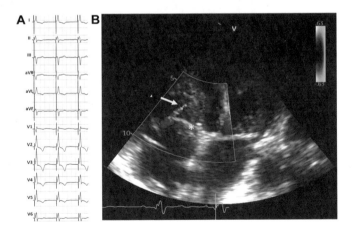

Figure 6-15   A: Successful left bundle branch area pacing (LBBAP); B: TTE showed septal CAF (yellow arrow) toward RV, due to LBBAP screw attempts. The final LBBAP lead position could be seen at the basal septum (yellow asterisk).

According to the position of fistula drainage, CAF can be divided into 5 types:

—Type Ⅰ drainage into RA;

—Type Ⅱ drainage into RV;

—Type Ⅲ drainage into PA;

—Type Ⅳ drainage into LA;

—Type Ⅴ drainage into LV.

Wearn classification of CAF can be seen in Figure 6-16.

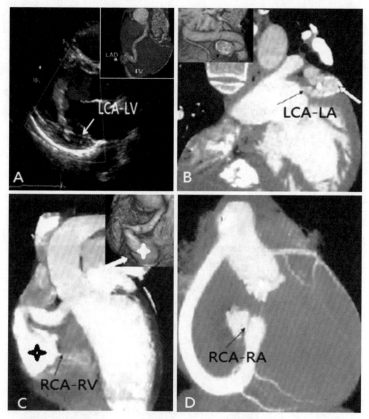

Figure 6-16 A: Echo showed LCA-LV fistula; B: CT image showed LCA-LA fistula with dilated RCA; C & D: CT images showed RCA-RV fistula and RCA-RA fistula with AN.

—Type Ⅰ is the arterial-cardiac fistula, in which the coronary artery is directed into the cardiac cavity;

—Type Ⅱ is the arterial-sinus fistula, in which the coronary artery communicates with the sinus network;

—Type Ⅲ is the arterial-capillary fistula, in which the coronary artery is injected into the capillary, and communicates with the cardiac cavity through the Thebesius system (small cardiac vein).

Yuksel S analyzed the angiographic data of 16,573 patients (Tables 6-2, 6-3) and found only 15 cases of CCF (0.09%), 8 males and 7 females, with an average age of 63 ± 12 years.

Table 6-2   Distribution of fistula origin sites in 15 patients with CCF

Origin	Patients, n	Angiographic prevalence, %	Anomaly prevalence, %
LAD artery	7	0.42	46.6
LCX artery	3	0.018	20
RCA	2	0.012	13.3
RCA and LCX artery	1	0.006	6.7
LAD artery and RCA	1	0.006	6.7
LAD artery, LCX artery, and RCA	1	0.006	6.7

Table 6-3   Distribution of fistula sites in 15 patients with CCF

Site of drainage	Patients, n	Angiographic prevalence, %	Anomaly prevalence, %
RV	4	0.024	27
LV	4	0.024	27
LA	4	0.024	27
RA	2	0.012	12
PA	1	0.006	7

Benoy N initially presented a highly unusual case with AN, the largest of which expanded further into RA, thus creating CCF (Figures 6-17, 6-18).

Leire U reported the percutaneous closure of giant CAF in an adult patient with angina and previous pericardiectomy (Figures 6-19, 6-20).

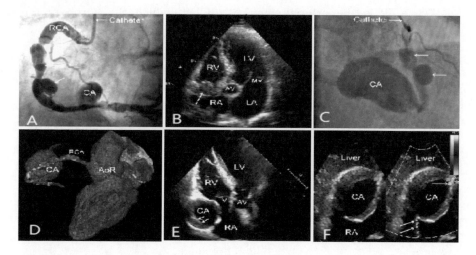

Figure 6-17　A: Diffusely ectatic RCA with several AN (white arrows); B: Echo visualized the distal AN adjacent to the right coronary sulcus (arrow); C: Huge expansion of the most distal AN on repeat angiography a decade later; D: 3-D CT reconstruction showed RCA and associated AN; E: Echo clearly delineated AN with mural thrombus; F: CDFI confirmed continuous flow from AN into RA (white arrows).

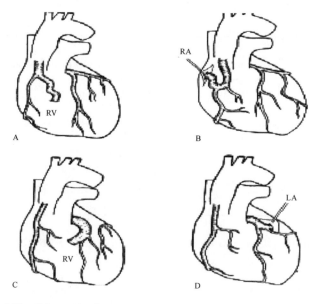

Figure 6-18　Schematic diagram of various CCF types. A: RCA-RV fistula; B: RCA-RA fistula; C: LCA-RV fistula; D: LCA-LA fistula.

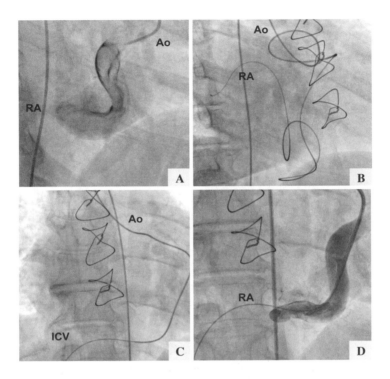

Figure 6-19   A: Coronary angiogram showed the fistula with drainage in RA; B: Advance of hydrophilic wire through the fistulous vessel to RA; C: Arteriovenous loop reaching the inferior vein cava; D: Selective ICA of the fistula from the aortic side.

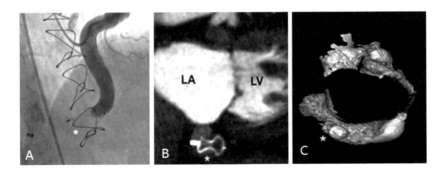

Figure 6-20   A: Percutaneous closure of the fistula; B & C: CT showed the Amplatzer duct occluder (asterisk) at the mouth of the fistula.

One case with multiple CAF was hospitalized due to paroxysmal chest pain for 2 days. ECG showed sinus rhythm and mild ST-T changes in precordial leads. No obvious abnormality of cardiac structure and function was found in Echo. Coronary angiogram showed no apparent stenosis in LAD, LCX and RCA. However, a slender vascular plexus issued from the near middle part of LAD and drained to LA, the distal end of LCX also issued a slender vascular plexus to the great cardiac vein, and a tortuous vessel issued from the opening of RCA to PA. (Figure 6-21).

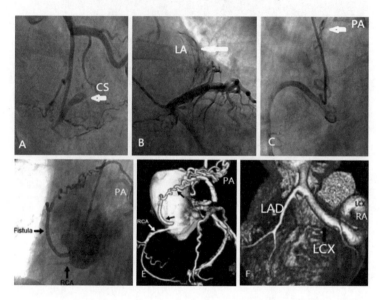

Figure 6-21 Angiogram of multiple CAF. A: LCX-CS fistula; B: LAD-LA fistula; C: RCA-PA fistula; D & E: Angiogram and CT image of right coronary sinus-PA fistula, and LCX-PA fistula was also found (E); F: LCX-RA fistula.

Ogden JA classified coronary artery-LA fistula into 3 types:

—Type Ⅰ: a short and thick fistula originating from LM or LCX entering LAA;

—Type Ⅱ: originating from the sinus node branch of any coronary artery;

—Type Ⅲ: fistula terminates on the posterior surface of LA along with the atrioventricular sulcus.

Sakakibara S and others classified the abnormal CAF into 3 types according to the dilated part (Figure 6-22):

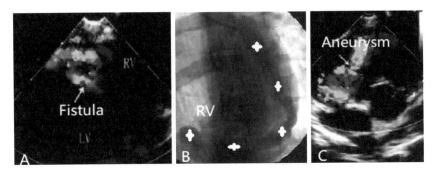

Figure 6-22   A: Fistula ostium; B: LCA-RV fistula with dilated RCA;
C: RCA aneurysm.

—Type Ⅰ (most common): a branch of LM showed tumor-like expansion;

　—Type Ⅱ: dilation of the initial and middle coronary artery;

　—Type Ⅲ: whole coronary artery dilatation.

Skalleberg ADL divided CAF into 6 types according to the fistula origin (Figure 6-23):

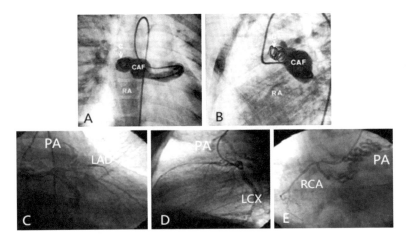

Figure 6-23   A & B: Angiogram of coronary artery-RA fistula (A, pre-TCC and B, post-TCC); C & E: Angiogram of 3 main CAPF with AMI.

　—RCA fistula;

　—LCA fistula;

　—Single CAF;

—Multiple CAF;

—Accessory CAF;

—There is no specific origin of coronary artery.

A large number of clinical data showed that the diameter of the involved vessel of CAF varies greatly, with only about 2 mm in the small and more than 20 mm in the large; the size of the involved vessel is so different that the choice of treatment methods is bound to be various. Some scholars have divided CAF into 3 types according to the diameter of involved vessels (Figure 6-24):

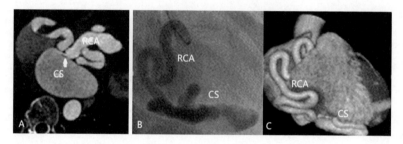

Figure 6-24   CT images (A, C) and angiogram (B) of RCA dilatation with small RCA-CS fistula.

—the diameter of involved vessel ≤ 5 mm is small and fine;

—the diameter of the involved vessel ≥ 10 mm is huge;

—the intermediate type (from 5 mm to 10 mm).

Dai Q retrospectively analyzed the imaging data of 21 patients with CAF who underwent CTA and confirmed the diagnosis after VR, MPR, MIP and CPR. The results showed that:

(1) among the fistula branches, 12 cases had single fistula, including 4 cases originating from RCA and 8 cases from LCA; multiple fistulas in 9 cases; the fistula was drained to PA in 16 cases, to LA in 1 case, and 2 cases to RA and LV respectively.

(2) The fistula artery showed dilation, tortuosity, or only vascular plexus. 2 cases were complicated with AN, 1 case with pericardial effusion and 1 case with LV aneurysm, and none of them was complicated with other intracardiac malformations.

(3) 17 cases were confirmed by ICA, and 7 cases underwent surgery. The authors believe that CTA can noninvasively and accurately display the origin, course, drainage site and combined abnormalities of CAF (Figures 6-25, 6-26, and 6-27).

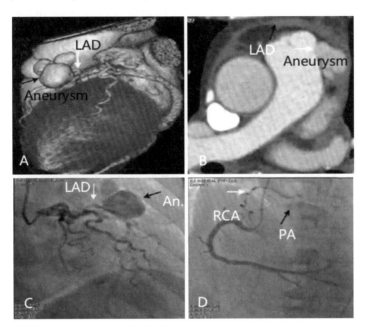

Figure 6-25 CT images and angiogram of multiple CAF. A-C: LAD-PA fistula with AN; D: RCA-PA fistula.

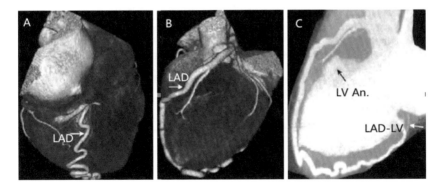

Figure 6-26 CT images of single LAD-LV fistula.

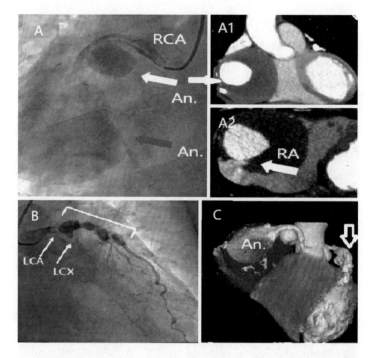

Figure 6-27   A: ICA showed 2 giant RCA aneurysms (white and red arrows); A1: CT image showed an 85 mm round mass in RCA; A2: RCA aneurysm ruptured into RA (white arrow); B & C: Severe LM stenosis (> 90%), an occluded LCX (white arrows) and multiple CAF in LM and the proximal portion of LAD (white rectangle).

Li W retrospectively summarized 9,000 patients who underwent CTA, and counted the incidence and imaging manifestations of CAF. The results found 23 cases of CAF, 20 cases of fistula were located in PA, 1 case in LAA, 1 case in LV and 1 case in CS. The authors believe that CTA combined with various reconstruction methods can show the origin, course and termination of CAF in the whole process, which is of great value in diagnosing congenital CAF (Figure 6-28).

It also can be divided into 2 types according to the presence or absence of other intracardiac malformations:

—isolated (simple, single) CAF accounts for about 80% of congenital CAF;

—secondary (complex, composite) CAF accounts for about 20% of

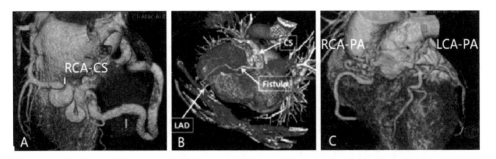

Figure 6-28   A: RCA-CS fistula with dilated RCA; B: LAD-CS fistula;
C: RCA/LCA-PA fistula.

congenital CAF.

Danzi GB reported a case of simple (isolated) CAF with myocardial
ischemia blocked by coil (Figure 6-29).

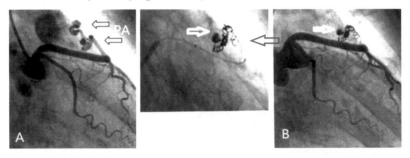

Figure 6-29   Angiogram before and after coil closure of LAD-PA fistula.

Pelleda GM and Bhat PSS reported 2 cases of TOF, VSD and CAF
(Figure 6-30).

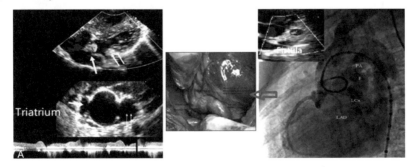

Figure 6-30   A: Echo of TOF with CAF; B: Angiogram of LCX-PA
fistula and surgical field.

In 1966, Sakakibara S divided CAF into 2 types according to the widened part of the coronary artery (Figures 6-31, 6-32):

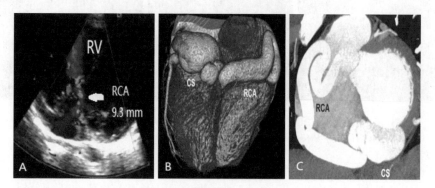

Figure 6-31 A: Echo of RCA-RV fistula, the red blood flow entered RV through the dilated RCA; B & C: CT images of RCA-CS fistula with RCA and CS dilated significantly.

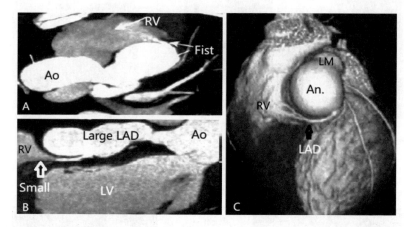

Figure 6-32 CT images of LM-RV fistula. A: The left sinus was enlarged, and LM and proximal fistula were significantly dilated; B: The middle segment of CAF was spherical, and the distal segment of CAF was thin; C: The distal end of CAF was opened in the anterior wall of RV, and the proximal segment of LAD was compressed and moved to the left.

—Type A (proximal type): The proximal coronary artery is widened, and the distal blood flow is normal. This CAF can be ligated in the epicardium.

—Type B (distal type): The whole coronary artery is widened, especially the dilated distal artery draining into the right heart system. This CAF can be sutured under CPB.

Yoshihara S and others reported a case of CAPF with multiple AN via Vieussens arterial ring (Figure 6-33).

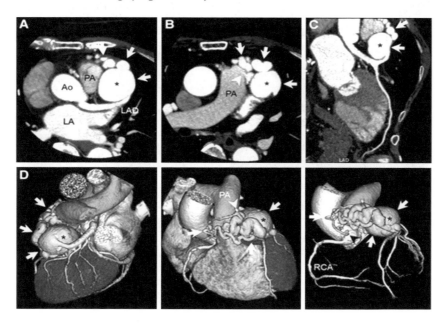

Figure 6-33   CTA of CAPF and AN. A-C: A large group of multiple tortuous serpiginous vessels with AN (arrows) arose from LAD, which drained into PA. The largest AN was 38 mm × 36 mm in diameter (asterisk). LM and proximal LAD are dilated. D: CTA showed CAF draining into the main PA with AN formation. Abnormal vessels also communicated with the conus artery arising separately from the right CS (black arrowhead), forming an aneurysmal Vieussens arterial ring.

Meta analysis showed that 20%–33.8% of patients could co-exist with other cardiovascular malformations. The distal and proximal openings of the fistula vary greatly, and the distal fistula is generally small. Calcification can be found in the wall of individual fistula. The ascending aorta is usually dilated to varying degrees, but it is not as obvious as that of PDA. Jux C and others reported several cases of CAF which depended on systemic perfusion and CCF with huge AN (Figure 6-34).

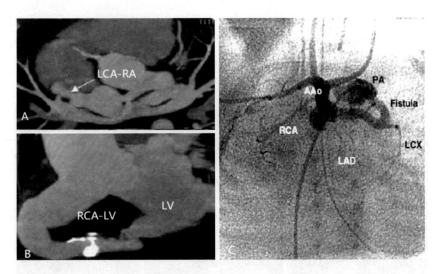

Figure 6-34   A: LCA-RA fistula. The left coronary sinus swelled, and the sinoatrial node branch of LCA expanded significantly, entering RA from the posterior superior wall. The distal segment of the thick sinoatrial node branch showed multiple tumor-like expansion; B: RCA-LV fistula. RCA was tumor-like dilated and entered LV; C: Angiographic changes of LCX-PA fistula.

Kim CY reported a rare case of CCF in which LCA and RCA joined together and drained into LV (Figure 6-35).

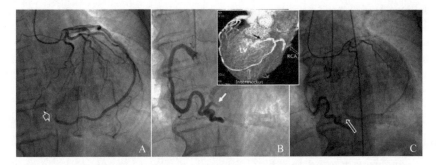

Figure 6-35   A: The arrow indicated the entering point from LAD; B: Angiogram showed tortuous RCA emptying into a certain cavity, and another artery (arrow) near the entering point; C: With simultaneous contrast injection, it was demonstrated that the intermedius and RCA joined together (arrow) and emptied into the cavity.

Chen K summarized case reports of aortocoronary arteriovenous fistula (ACAVF) after CABG. A total of 48 ACAVF cases post-CABG were gathered. Among these patients, the mean age was 61.9 years, and 79.2% were men. The most common presenting symptoms were chest pain (60.4%) and dyspnea (27.1%). The average time of initial symptoms was 3 years. However, 54.2% of patients developed symptoms within the first year. The most involved vessel was LAD during CABG (62.5%). Of these cases, 9 (18.8%) were managed conservatively, 8 (16.7%) chose to undergo surgery, including ligation of fistula and CABG, and 27 (56.3%) underwent percutaneous closure. Among these patients, 13 cases (27.1%) were managed with coil embolization, 5 (10.4%) with balloon embolization, 5 (10.4%) were treated with a covered stent, and 4 (8.3%) used AVP. There were no reported complications following treatment in this group.

Inadvertent ACAVF is rare following CABG. The differential diagnosis for recurrent angina or exertional dyspnea after CABG should include inadvertent ACAVF formation, in addition to the more common reasons like graft degeneration or disease progression in the native vessels. If untreated, ACAVF can lead to serious complications. Cardiac catheterization remains the gold standard for diagnosis, although MDCT has the potential to be as effective with less risk and cost. Asymptomatic patients can be managed conservatively, although the majority of patients are symptomatic on presentation. Redoing CABG or surgical ligation of the fistula requires repeat thoracotomy, and percutaneous interventions with coil or balloon embolization are associated with the risks of thrombosis and distal embolization. Using covered stents and AVP has proven to be plausible and practical alternative options. Percutaneous closure is feasible and safe in treating these patients (Figure 6-36).

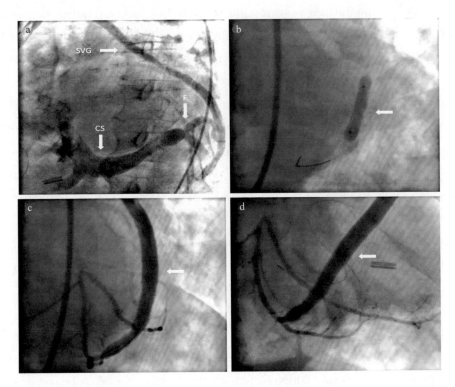

Figure 6-36   Cardiac catheterization of an 81-year-old patient with a previous history of CABG. (a) There was a fistula (F) between the saphenous vein graft (SVG) and CS; (b) A stent was deployed (arrow); (c) A balloon was used to expand the stent (arrow); (d) ACAVF was successfully occluded.

Kanzaki T reported a case with CAVF draining into PLSVC, and performed closure of the fistula, and CABG. Post-operative CTA showed patency of all the grafts and progression of thrombosis in the dilated abnormal vessels (Figures 6-37, 6-38).

Sunkara A and others presented several cases with multiple CAF with significant hemodynamic consequences (Figures 6-39, 6-40, 6-41, 6-42, and 6-43).

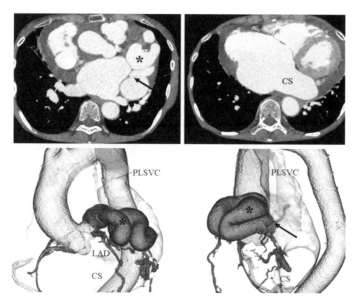

Figure 6-37   Post-operative CTA: CAVF (arrow) originating from LCX and draining into PLSVC (* dilated LM and LCX).

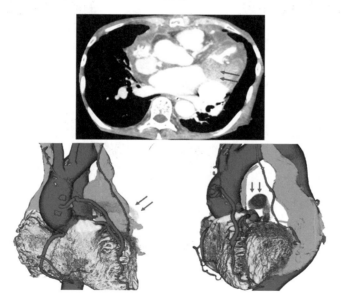

Figure 6-38   Post-operative CTA: Progression of thrombosis (arrows) in LCX and CAVF. All grafts are patent.

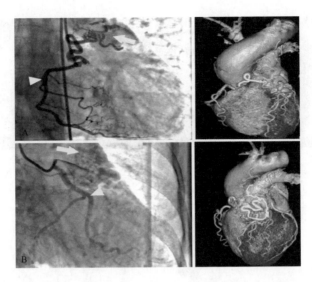

Figure 6-39 A: ICA showed fistula (arrow) of RCA (arrowhead). CTA showed fistula (yellow line) from RCA to PA; B: ICA showed fistula (arrow) of LAD (arrowhead). CTA showed fistula (yellow line) from LAD to PA.

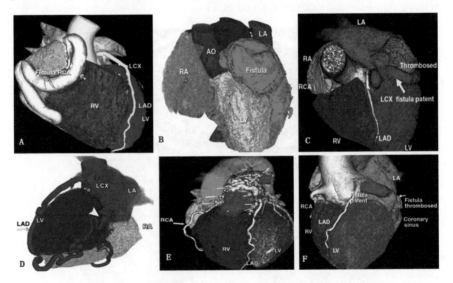

Figure 6-40 MDCT of RCA-RA fistula (A), LM and LCX-RA fistula (B), TCC for LCX-CS fistula and had a partial recurrence of fistula at 5-year follow-up evaluation (C), LAD-LV fistula detected during evaluation of occasional chest pain and cardiac murmur, fistulous connections (arrows) from LAD and RCA to PA (E), and new-onset chest pain due to thrombus in residual CAF and history of coil embolization for LCX-CS fistula.

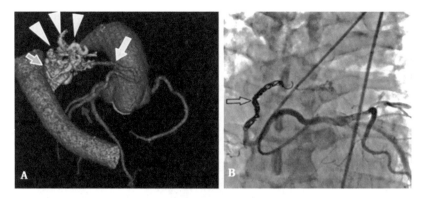

Figure 6-41   Coronary-bronchial artery fistula that resulted in likely coronary steal phenomenon and was treated with coil embolization. A: MDCT showed large collateral vessel (yellow arrow) originating from LCX (red arrow) to the bronchial collateral network (yellow arrowheads) and connecting to an intercostal artery (blue arrow); B: Embolization using the Penumbra coils (green arrow).

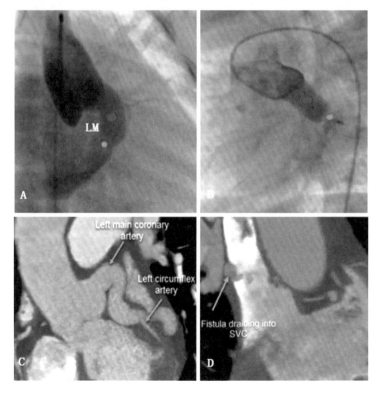

Figure 6-42   LM fistula with aortic steal phenomenon, CHF and arrest. A & B: Pre- and post-TCC of LM fistula; C & D: LM-SVC fistula.

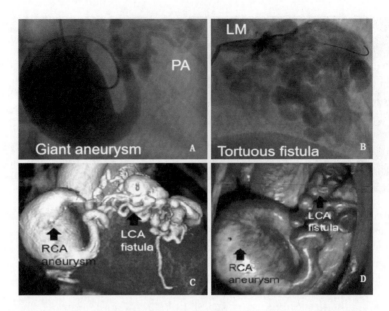

Figure 6-43   A: ICA showed a giant aneurysm originating from RCA and draining into PA; B: LCA with a tortuous fistula and drainage to PA near the ostial segment of LAD; C: MDCT showed RCA-PA fistula and LAD-PA fistula with giant AN; D: Surgical image of the giant AN and torturous fistula.

Chapter VII Clinical manifestations

Highlights

- Most of the clinical manifestations of CAF are atypical, and many CAF have no obvious symptoms. However, larger CAF can be accompanied by clinical symptoms, such as palpitation, chest tightness, and dyspnea.

- With age, the symptoms gradually worsen, and CHF may occur. Myocardial ischemia or AMI and IE are the serious complications of CAF. Thrombosis can be formed in AN, and thrombus shedding can cause distal coronary embolism. AN can also compress adjacent coronary arteries, affecting the blood supply of the myocardium, and AN can even rupture and produce serious complications.

- The incidence of symptoms and complications in patients with CAF after the age of 20 is 55% and 35%, but that before the age of 20 is 9% and 11%, respectively.

- The murmur of CAF is mostly continuous, and the loudest in diastole; fistula into LV is diastolic murmur.

- The occurrence time of symptoms in patients with CAF is closely related to the volume of shunt flow, the abnormal location of fistula, and other congenital cardiovascular malformations. The incidence of CAF complications also increases with age.

- CAP is an uncommon but potentially severe complication of PCI, and is observed most frequently in complex procedures. Clinical outcomes, including periprocedural and long-term mortality, are markedly worse with increasing perforation. Perforation which requires covered stent usage predicts a high in-hospital and overall mortality, although no difference is noted with covered stent type.

CAF has various manifestations. Some determinants of severity are the origin, termination site, length, and size of the fistula. However, despite this, most patients with CAF have no symptoms. Generally speaking, fistula had no symptoms for about 20 years. Only 19% of patients had symptoms before the age of 20, and 63% had symptoms of different degrees after the age of 20; 59% of the patients were asymptomatic before the age of 20, and only 21.8% after the age of 20. Yildiz BS reported a 65-year-old case of coronary artery-LV fistula with apical hypertrophic cardiomyopathy and unstable angina (Figure 7-1).

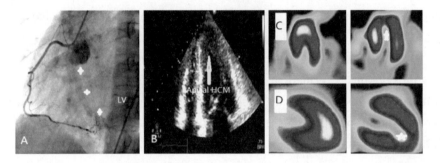

Figure 7-1   A: RCA-LV fistula (asterisk); B: Apical hypertrophic cardiomyopathy (yellow arrow); C & D: ECT images showed myocardial ischemia (asterisk).

However, symptoms and signs will appear once the fistula begins to become hemodynamically significant. Grade 2-3/6 continuous murmur with local tremors can be heard in the precordial area, and the loudest part of the murmur depends on the drainage site where the CAF enters the heart. In the case of RV fistula, the 4th and 5th intercostal diastolic murmur at the left edge of sternum was the loudest, while in the case of fistula into RA, the 2nd intercostal systolic murmur at the right edge of the sternum was the loudest. The murmur of PA or LA fistula is the loudest along the 2nd intercostal space at the left edge of the sternum (Figure 7-2). Cardiac murmur is found during physical examination, but those with large left-right shunt flow may have symptoms of palpitation, angina and CHF. If the fistula enters RA, it is more likely to have CHF symptoms, and the fistula into CS is prone to atrial fibrillation (Figure 7-3).

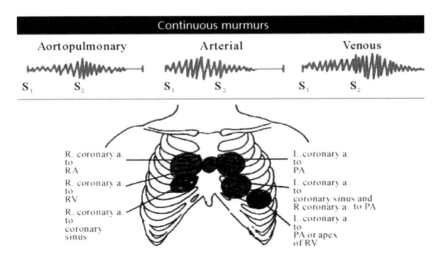

Figure 7-2 Schematic diagram of murmur and auscultation area of CAF.

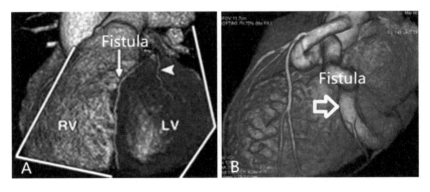

Figure 7-3 A: The small CAF with no symptoms; B: The huge CAF with CHF.

The followings are some common manifestations of CAF:

—Congenital CAF: In infants aged 3-4 months, a hemodynamically significant CAF may manifest as CHF. Babies have tachycardia, shortness of breath, and are usually irritable, restless and sweating. Continuous murmurs can be heard during cardiac auscultation. In general, if the dilated coronary artery is more than 3 times larger than normal, symptoms will occur. Many patients with CAF have a small fistula, usually without clinical symptoms when young, and only occasionally found in ICA. In adulthood, most of them usually seek medical treatment because of dyspnea, chest pain, and arrhythmia.

—Asymptomatic adult patients: Most patients with CAF remain asymptomatic for at least 10 or 20 years. Physical examination occasionally reveals persistent murmurs, which are usually best heard in the precordial area. Most fistulas are found by accident during ICA.

—AMI or chronic myocardial ischemia: CAF affects the myocardium through the coronary steal phenomenon. In this case, the blood vessels at the distal end of CAF do not receive enough blood, so the area they supply will be ischemic. Another mechanism of myocardial ischemia caused by fistula is thrombosis at the junction of normal and abnormal coronary arteries, and the patient may have typical or atypical chest pain. However, in some cases, patients may experience persistent chronic pain and don't improve after rest.

Jang SN reported a case of double coronary arteries-RV fistula with variant angina pectoris (Figure 7-4). Majidi M reported a 44-year-old patient with chest pain, AMI, CHF, and VT. During ICA, LAD-PA fistula was found (Figure 7-5).

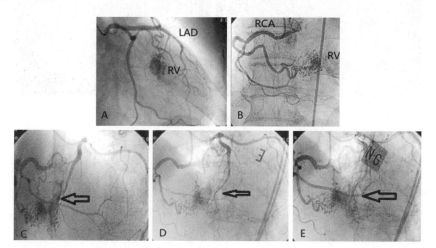

Figure 7-4   A & B: Angiogram showed double coronary artery-RV fistula; C-E: Angiogram before and after Ergotamine provocation test. Before Ergotamine injection (C), angina and diffuse stenosis of LAD occurred after Ergotamine injection (D), the symptoms were relieved and the degree of stenosis was reduced after Nitroglycerin injection (E).

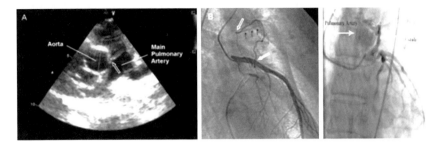

Figure 7-5   A & B: Echo and angiogram showed LAD-PA fistula; C: Another case with LAD-PA fistula.

—CHF: CAF with a large left-right shunt can lead to pulmonary volume overload, which may prompt the symptoms of right heart failure. The patient may have shortness of breath, chest discomfort, and pitting edema. Above are the most common manifestations in patients with congenital fistula, which usually occurs in infancy and childhood. Left and/or right CHF can occur due to different degrees of cardiac chamber overload, with an incidence of 18.3%. It is easy to occur in infants and after the age of 20, especially in patients aged 40-50 who need to engage in heavy physical labor.

When multiple fistula orifices of CAF exist, a sponge-like vascular plexus can be formed. CAF draining into the right cardiac cavity can lead to pulmonary volume overload and pulmonary hypertension; CAF draining into LV can lead to volume overload and LV hypertrophy. CHF can be caused by the long course of the disease, gradual expansion of fistula, increase of shunt flow, and aggravation of cardiac load.

CHF is often caused by various diseases in that the myocardial contractility is weakened so that the blood output of the heart is reduced, which is not enough to meet the needs of the body, and then a series of symptoms and signs are produced. Left heart failure is mainly manifested by fatigue and dyspnea. At first, it is dyspnea on exertion, and finally, it evolves into dyspnea at rest and orthopnea or paroxysmal nocturnal dyspnea. It has chest tightness, shortness of breath, cough, and wheezing, and serious cases can evolve into acute pulmonary edema with severe asthma, extreme anxiety, cough with foam mucus sputum (typically pink frothy sputum), cyanosis and other symptoms of pulmonary congestion. The main manifestations of right heart failure are edema of lower limbs, jugular vein distention, loss of appetite, nausea and vomiting, oliguria, nocturia, separation of drinking water and urination, etc.

Osranek M reported a 31-year-old female patient with dyspnea on exertion and cardiac murmur at birth. Echo examination found LCA-RA fistula (Figure 7-6A). Mullens W reported a case of CAF with right heart failure (Figures 7-6B and C).

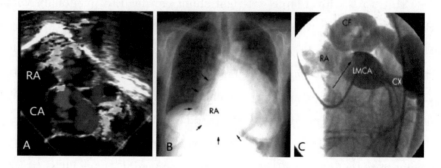

Figure 7-6　A: Echo of LCA-RA fistula; B: Chest X-ray film of CAF with right heart failure and enlargement of RA; C: Angiogram of LCX-RA fistula with dilated LM and LCX.

—Atrial and ventricular arrhythmia: The mechanism of arrhythmia with CAF is low cardiac output and blood flow reserve, followed by atrial and/or ventricular dilation.

—Cardiac tamponade: Although rare, in some cases, rupture of CAF may lead to pericardial hematocele. This will lead to shortness of breath, hypotension, jugular vein distention, and abnormal pulse. Harada Y reported a special case of spontaneous rupture of CAF, pericardial tamponade and sudden death (Figure 7-7).

—Pulmonary hypertension: It is often seen in patients with CAF flowing into the right cardiac cavity, blood vessel, or coronary sinus. Severe patients may have dyspnea or even serious complications such as secondary polycythemia, IE, dilated vascular rupture, and thrombosis.

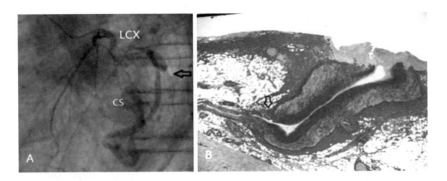

Figure 7-7   Angiogram and pathological changes of LCX-CS fistula.
A & B: Rupture of LCX (arrow).

—Subacute bacterial endocarditis (SBE) or IE: 2.5% – 10% of CAF cases can be complicated with SBE/IE. Bacterial endocarditis occurs when bacteria (microorganisms) enter the bloodstream and lodge on the endocardial surface of the heart, and multiply in large numbers to cause infection. Ahn DS reported a case of RCA-LV fistula with mitral SBE (Figure 7-8).

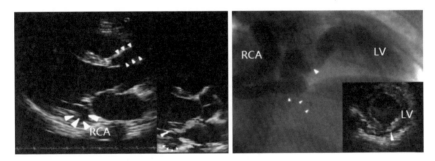

Figure 7-8   Echo and angiogram of RCA-LV fistula.

—Steal (ischemic) cardiomyopathy: Nearly 1/5 of patients can develop stable or unstable angina, usually middle-aged and elderly patients, often when they are active or tired, of which about 4% of patients can eventually develop AMI and endanger their lives. We reported a 41-year-old male patient with CAF and CHF for the first time globally. It was confirmed by pre- and post-operative Echo and ICA that the patient was a case of coronary steal induced cardiomyopathy caused by LCA-PA fistula (Figure 7-9).

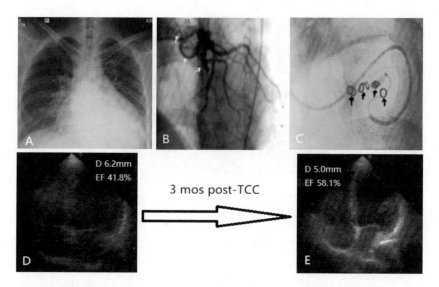

Figure 7-9 A: Chest X-ray film showed general cardiac enlargement;
B & C: Pre- and post-TCC; D&E: Echo pre- and post-TCC.

Most of the manifestations of patients with CAF are usually secondary to complications. The followings are possible complications caused by CAF:

—Steal syndrome: Blood is shunted through a fistula, resulting in a decrease in distal blood flow and myocardial ischemia;

—Thrombosis or embolism: causes AMI;

—Volume overload: causes CHF and arrhythmia;

—Rupture: causes hemopericardium and pericardial tamponade;

—Endocarditis or endarteritis.

On physical examination, there are no pertinent findings. However, a continuous murmur may be auscultated, which can be confused with PDA. The murmur of CAF is heard lower on the left sternal border, which is not the typical location for PDA. The large left-left shunt may cause a widened mean arterial pressure (MAP), as is commonly seen with significant aortic regurgitation.

Meta analysis showed that children with CAF were mostly asymptomatic (80%), while about 40% of adults shared symptoms of fatigue, dyspnea, angina, and CHF (Table 7-1).

Table 7-1   The frequency (%) of CAF symptoms presentation

Symptoms	Frequency (cases %)
Dyspnea	Common (60%)
Endocarditis	Good (20%)
Congestive heart failure	Good (19%)
Angina	Moderate (3%－7%)
Syncope	Uncommon
Palpitation	Uncommon
Cardiac arrhythmia	Uncommon
Hemopericardium	Rare
Cardiac tamponade	Rare
Sudden cardiac death	Isolated

Malik M reported a patient presenting with chest pain diagnosed with NSTEMI and noted CAF on subsequent investigations. This case highlights the initial medical management of NSTEMI and the subsequent management of CAF (Figure 7-10).

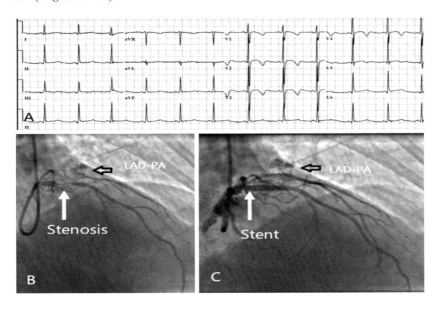

Figure 7-10   A: ECG showed anterolateral T wave inversion; B: Large LAD-PA fistula arising from stenotic segment; C: After PCI.

Kemmochi R reported an 82-year-old woman with a history of rest angina and palpitations. ECG revealed no signs of ischemia but exhibited atrial fibrillation. Chest X-ray showed cardiomegaly and pulmonary congestion. Coronary angiogram revealed giant AN arising from LCX but did not provide detailed information. MDCT revealed dilated and tortuous LCA with a 40 mm AN. The distal side drained into CS. Surgery was performed to close the fistula and seclude all parts of the aneurysmal coronary artery. All coronary branches emerging from AN required bypass grafting (Figure 7-11).

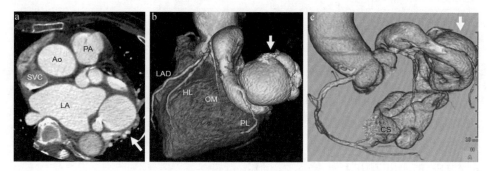

Figure 7-11 Pre-operative MDCT showed giant LCX aneurysm (arrows). LCA was dilated and tortuous for its entire length starting from the coronary ostium, and directly connected to CS.

The clinical manifestation of CAF mainly depends on the severity of the left-right shunt. Several studies have found that most adult cases have no symptoms, and on the contrary, children have more clinical symptoms, which may be due to the larger fistula in them. Children often seek medical treatment because of abnormal ECG and chest X-ray or continuous murmur. Boulmier D reported a 50-year-old asymptomatic female patient who found a huge RCA-RA fistula during ICA (Figure 7-12A). Manghat NE reported a 63-year-old patient with paroxysmal atrial fibrillation who failed drug therapy. CT examination showed a small LAD-pulmonary venous fistula (Figure 7-12B).

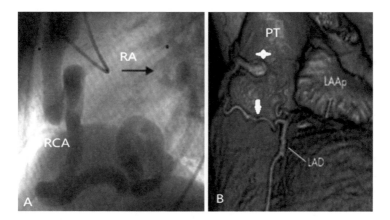

Figure 7-12 A: Angiogram showed RCA-RA fistula with no symptoms;
B: CT image showed LAD-pulmonary vein fistula with atrial fibrillation.

Chapter VIII Supplementary examination

Highlights

- Laboratory examination: There is no relevant data at present.
- ECG can show high LV voltage, LV or biventricular hypertrophy. If the fistula drains into RV, there is RV hypertrophy. Atrial fibrillation may be found in patients with shunt into RA. Although CAF has potential myocardial ischemia, it is rare to have ST-T changes in ECG.
- Echo examination can clearly show the direction of the coronary artery, including the origin and drainage site of CAF, and CDFI can find the location and shunt volume of the fistula.
- Cardiac catheterization showed high blood oxygen content in the shunted cardiac cavity, especially in RA, RV or PA, indicating the existence of left-right shunt. At the same time, the capacity of its shunt flow and PA pressure can be measured.
- Ascending aortic angiography should be the first choice, and selective ICA is needed for small CAF.

Examination items of CAF include ECG, chest X-ray, Echo, and CDFI, CT and MR, aortic angiography or ICA, and lab examination (Table 8-1).

The diagnosis of CAF mainly depends on imaging-related examinations, so the following focuses on radiology, Echo, and interventional examinations.

Chest X-ray can show the size of the heart, and those with aneurysmal dilatation of the coronary artery can change the contour of the heart; Echo can find the dilated coronary artery and the site of CAF into the cardiac cavity, which is easier to diagnose; cardiac catheterization can detect the increase of blood oxygen content; retrograde ascending aortic angiography and selective ICA can show the morphology of the involved coronary artery and the location of CAF, which are the basis for clear diagnosis and treatment plan; CTA or MR can show the shape, course and position of the involved coronary artery, which is an invaluable non-invasive examination method (Figures 8-1, 8-2, and 8-3).

Table 8-1   Advantages and limitations of various imaging modalities in CAF evaluation

Imaging Modality	Advantages	Limitations
ICA	Excellent spatial and temporal resolution Good hemodynamic information Good evaluation of the size and the number of fistulous tracts Diagnosis and treatment can be rendered at the same time	Catheter-related risks Two-dimensional fluoroscopic images can obscure complex anomalous vessels Radiation exposure Iodinated contrast material toxicity
Echo	No exposure to radiation Microbubble contrast material can improve identification of CAF and their course	Limited field of view can limit assessment of fistulous tracts and/or other extracardiac structures Operator dependency Poor Echo window
CTA	Good spatial and temporal resolution Short acquisition time Excellent anatomic information obtained by using 3-D multiplanar imaging with volume rendering Wide field of view enables evaluation of complex anatomy related to CAF	Radiation exposure Iodinated contrast material toxicity Less hemodynamic information
MR angiography	Noninvasive No exposure to radiation No contrast material needed	Lower spatial resolution and contrast-to-noise ratio Long acquisition time Less clear information regarding the fistulous origin and drainage site (compared with information acquired with CTA or ICA)

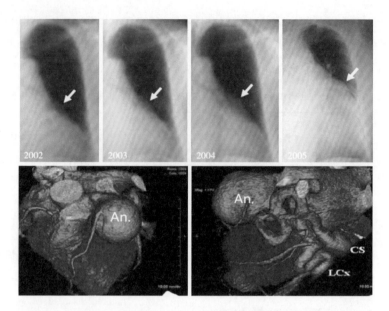

Figure 8-1 Serial chest X-ray films and CT images of LM-CS fistula.

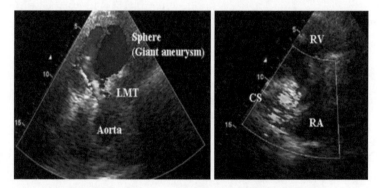

Figure 8-2 Echo of LM-CS fistula with huge AN.

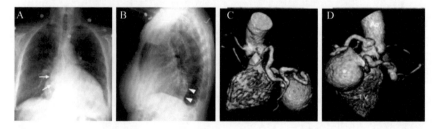

Figure 8-3 Chest X-ray films and CT images of LCX-CS fistula. A & B: Cardiac enlargement; C & D: LCX-CS fistula with huge AN.

Ahmad T and others reported several cases of giant AN with RCA-RA fistula (Figures 8-4, 8-5).

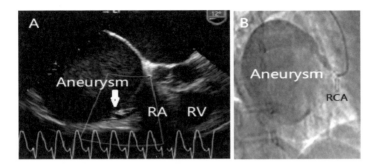

Figure 8-4   Echo and angiogram of RCA-RA fistula with huge AN.

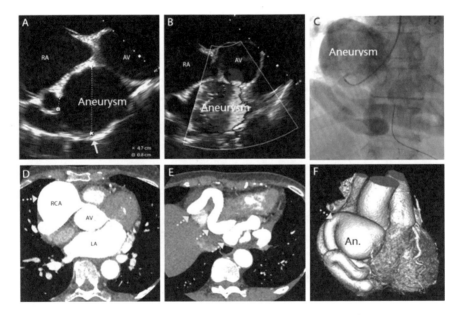

Figure 8-5   A: TEE showed a large aneurysmal structure (yellow arrow) adjacent to RA and aorta valve (47 mm in diameter) with turbulent flow on CDFI (B); C: ICA demonstrated a large RCA aneurysm proximally and a grossly ectatic vessel; D & E: CTA confirmed a large proximal RCA aneurysm (yellow interrupted arrow) with the remainder of the ectatic vessels and tortuous course (yellow interrupted arrow); F: CTA of RCA aneurysm (yellow interrupted arrow).

Section I ECG

Commonly the ECG findings are normal, or there may be evidence of LV volume overload and myocardial ischemia. In the older patient with coronary artery-RA fistula, atrial fibrillation may be present. CAF could lead to different degrees of the atrioventricular block due to ischemic changes or embryological pathways. However, most CAF are asymptomatic, and atrioventricular conduction abnormalities related to CAF are rare (Figures 8-6, 8-7). Regular ECG check-ups should be recommended in patients with CAF.

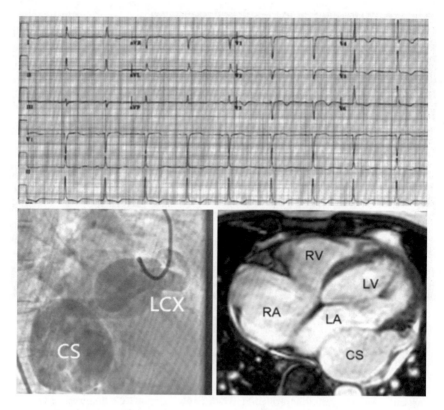

Figure 8-6 ECG showed Q wave formation, T wave inversion; angiogram and CTA showed LCX-CS fistula.

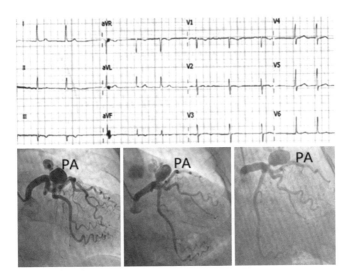

Figure 8-7   ECG and ICA of LCA-PA fistula. ECG showed T wave inversion
in precordial leads; Angiogram showed LCA-PA fistula with AN.

Yuksel M reported a case of 3 coronary arteries-LV fistula with atrial
fibrillation and angina pectoris (Figure 8-8).

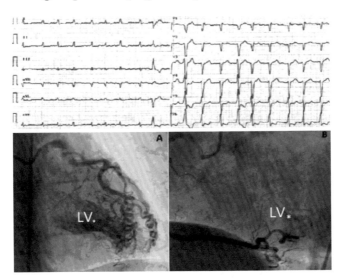

Figure 8-8   ECG and angiogram of 3 coronary arteries-LV
fistula with atrial fibrillation.

Mori K reported a case of double coronary arteries-RA fistula. During the follow-up, atrioventricular block and myocardial ischemia occurred (Figure 8-9).

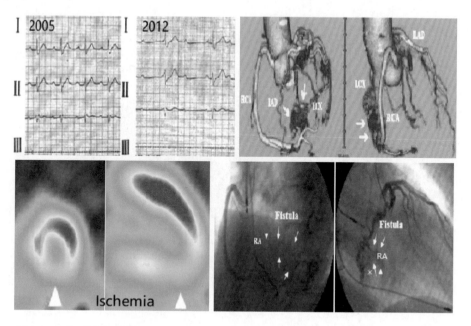

Figure 8-9 ECG, ECT and angiogram of CAF. Normal ECG in 2005 and complete atrioventricular block in 2012; ECT showed myocardial ischemia; ICA showed double coronary arteries-RA fistula.

Fan H reported a 67-year-old female patient who was admitted to hospital with frequent ventricular premature beats (VPB). Imaging examination found LAD-PA fistula with tumor-like expansion. After the successful operation, VPB disappeared (Figure 8-10).

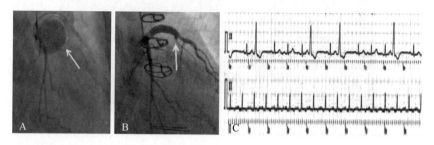

Figure 8-10 Angiographic changes of LAD-PA fistula before (A) and after (B) surgery. ECG showed that VPB disappeared after operation.

Although CAF has potential myocardial ischemia, it is rare to find ST-T changes and T wave inversion in ECG (Figure 8-11).

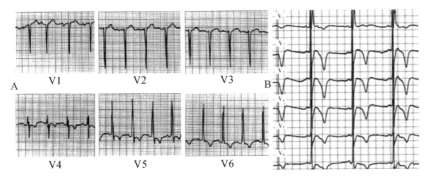

Figure 8-11   A: ECG of coronary artery-LV fistula with myocardial ischemia showed LV hypertrophy and T wave inversion in lead V4-V6; B: LAD-LV fistula with T wave inversion in lead V1-V6.

Section Ⅱ   Chest X-ray

—Coronary artery-right heart system or PA fistula belongs to left-right shunt in terms of hemodynamics. According to the X-ray findings, the pulmonary blood flow can increase in varying degrees, generally mild to moderate. The enlargement of the heart is mainly in LV, often accompanied by the enlargement of LA or RV, and the ascending aortic arch is often bulging (Figure 8-12).

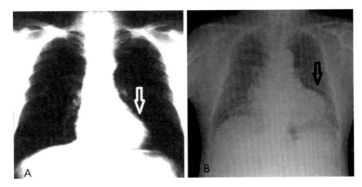

Figure 8-12   Chest X-ray films of coronary artery-RV fistula with RV hypertrophy and right heart failure. A: 16-year-old male; B: 58-year-old male.

—Coronary artery-left cardiac cavity fistula shows no sign of pulmonary congestion. Coronary artery-LV fistula is equivalent to aortic regurgitation in hemodynamics. The heart with the larger shunt flow is mostly aortic type, LV is increased from medium to large scale, the ascending aortic arch is swollen, and the heartbeat is enhanced, presenting a collapsed pulse (Figures 8-13, 8-14).

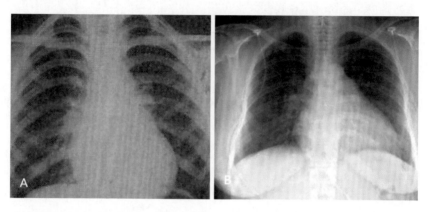

Figure 8-13　Chest X-ray films of coronary artery-LV fistula with cardiac enlargement. A: 25-year-old patient; B: 68-year-old patient.

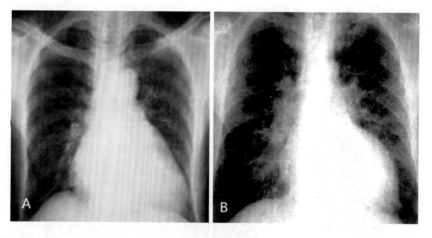

Figure 8-14　Chest X-ray films of coronary artery-LV fistula with LV hypertrophy and left heart failure. A: 14-year-old patient; B: 76-year-old patient.

—In some cases, the tortuous and dilated coronary artery (especially the right side) can form the edge of the heart shadow or an abnormal bulge.

Calcification can be seen in the dilated aneurysmal coronary arteries in a few cases (Figure 8-15).

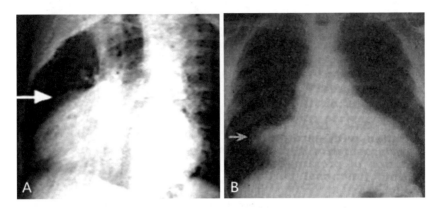

Figure 8-15   Chest X-ray films of RCA-RA fistula and RCA-LV fistula.

—Results of chest radiographs are usually normal, but there may be cardiomegaly or evidence of CHF.

Lee SY reported a geriatric patient with asymptomatic CAF that was incidentally found by chest radiography (Figure 8-16).

Chest X-ray film has some limitations in diagnosing CAF, and its specific sign is the abnormal pulsation and bulging shadow of the heart. This shadow is an abnormally dilated tortuous coronary artery. Combined with clinical murmur, it can preliminarily diagnose the disease, but the detection rate of this sign is low. In addition, the lung blood flow and LV, RV changes shown in the chest X-ray film are also helpful for diagnosing of CAF (Figure 8-17).

Xu Z analyzed and evaluated the clinical value of chest X-ray film and angiography in diagnosing congenital CAF, and discussed the occurrence of the disease. Forty-three cases of congenital CAF confirmed by the operation were diagnosed by chest X-ray film and angiography, including 16 males and 27 females, with an average age of 15. The results showed that 5 of 43 cases were definitely diagnosed by chest X-ray film, and all cases were correctly diagnosed by angiography. Among them, 28 cases (65%) originated from RCA, 14 cases (32.6%) from LCA and 1 case (2.4%) from double coronary arteries; fistula into LV in 18 cases (42%), RA in 15 cases (35%), LV in 5

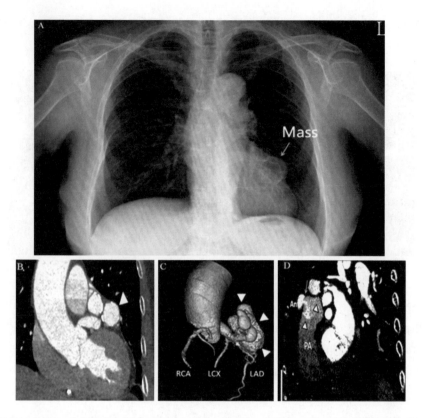

Figure 8-16 A: Chest X-ray film demonstrated a bulge with peripheral ring-like calcification on the left cardiac border (arrow); B: CT image showed multiple AN with calcified plaques (arrowhead); C: CTA displayed a fistula from LAD with multiple intervening AN (arrowheads); D: CT image demonstrated connecting channel (arrow) between aneurysmal fistula and PA. Patchy contrast medium jet was also displayed (arrowheads) within the pulmonary trunk.

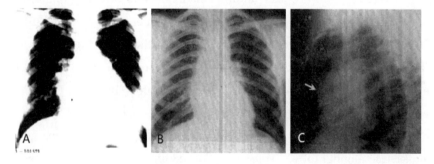

Figure 8-17 Chest X-ray films of multiple CAF with general heart enlargement (A) and RCA-RV fistula with local cardiac enlargement (B & C).

cases (12%), PA in 4 cases (9%), and LA in 1 case (2%). The authors believe that X-ray film has some limitations in diagnosing CAF. Still, it has a high diagnostic value if abnormal pulsation and local enlargement of the heart shadow are found.

Chest radiography can be used for follow-up after TCC or surgery operations (Figure 8-18).

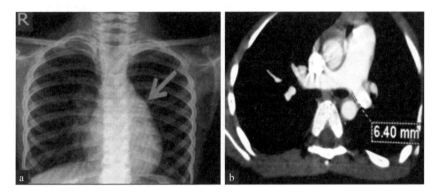

Figure 8-18   Chest X-ray film (a) and CTA image (b) of cardiac device in PA. Chest X-ray film revealed slight cardiomegaly and a device located in the left PA (a). CTA revealed dilated main PA, Amplatzer device located at 6.4mm from the bifurcation in the left PA (b) and distal PA showed normal contrast opacification.

Jeong EH and others analyzed the imaging changes of AN with CAF (Figures 8-19, 8-20).

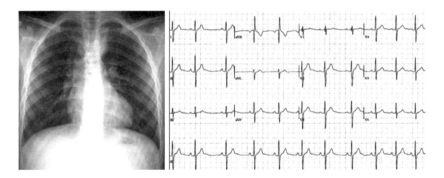

Figure 8-19   Chest X-ray and ECG of persistent AN and RCA-RV fistula.

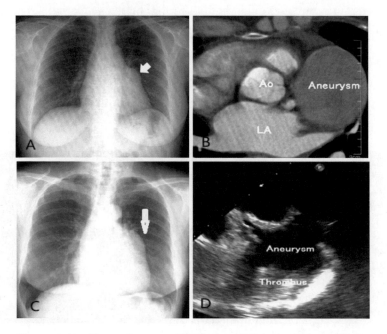

Figure 8-20   X-ray changes, CT image and Echo of AN with CAF.

Section Ⅲ   Echo

Echo has a high value in the diagnosis of CAF and is the most basic diagnostic method.

Echo characteristics of CAF: The most noticeable finding and direct sign is the significant expansion of the involved coronary artery with aneurysm-like changes. The fistula is generally long and tortuous; if the fistula is short, there may be no tortuous change. The blood flow signal in the coronary artery is enhanced, and the ejection and two-phase continuous blood flow appear in the heart cavity of CAF.

Two-dimensional Echo usually delineates the coronary anatomy, including where the fistula originates, which chamber it drains, and any chamber enlargement or hypertrophy. CDFI can also demonstrate the blood flow through the fistulous connection (Figures 8-21, 8-22, and 8-23).

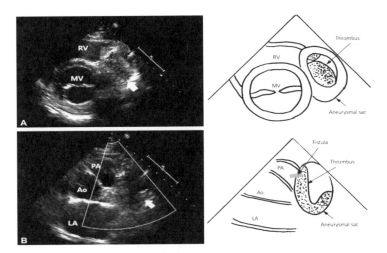

Figure 8-21 The parasternal short axis view of TTE. A: Aneurysmal sac (arrow) filled with thrombus, 4.1 cm × 4.0 cm in size; B: Fistula from the aneurysm to PA (color flow) and aneurysmal sac (arrow).

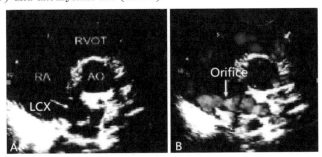

Figure 8-22 Echo characters of CAF. A: The tumor-like dilation of LCX; B: The location of fistula orifice.

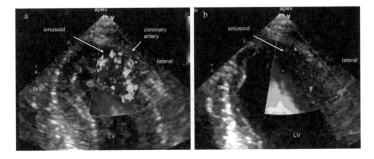

Figure 8-23 CDFI showed several tubular flow signals from the epicardium to LV chamber during diastole (a); During early systole, the opposite flow from LV lumen to the hypertrophic region was observed (b).

　　Sato K reported a scarce case of coronary artery-LV fistula through a sinusoid without cyanotic congenital heart disease or severe CAD (Figure 8-24). Li X reported a 44-year-old man with RCA-CS fistula diagnosed by three-dimensional Echo and confirmed by CTA and surgery (Figure 8-25).

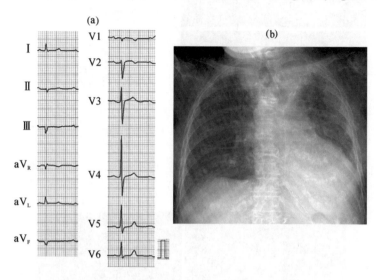

Figure 8-24　(a): ECG showed sinus rhythm with QS pattern in lead Ⅱ, Ⅲ, and aVF; (b): Chest X-ray showed pleural effusion.

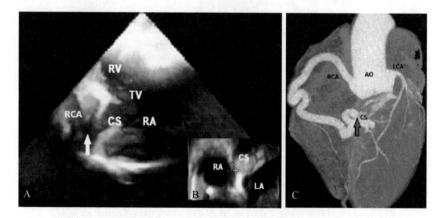

Figure 8-25　A: Echo showed the drainage site of CAF; B: The dilated RCA and CS; C: The black arrow showed the drainage site from RCA into CS.

Two-dimensional Echo and CDFI of CAF have some characteristic manifestations:

(1) The proximal segment of the involved coronary artery was dilated, significantly wider than the main coronary artery on the opposite side, and its course was tortuous and changeable. The fistula orifice can be found by tracing its course, and the atrioventricular wall is interrupted;

(2) CDFI showed abnormal blood flow signals at CAF course and fistula orifice. When the fistula enters the right heart system, it is the continuous turbulence spectrum of the whole cardiac cycle (Figure 8-26).

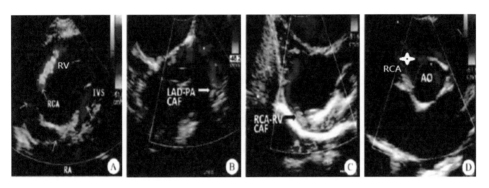

Figure 8-26   Echo findings of various CAF. A: RCA-RV fistula; B: LAD-PA fistula; C: RCA-RV fistula; D: The dilated RCA.

For children with good acoustic window conditions, TTE can obtain satisfactory image, and continuous biphasic murmur can be detected at the fistula. Contrast enhanced Echo with microbubbles helps determine the location, width and shunt flow of CAF. However, diagnosing CAF by TTE has great limitations, and the blood flow signals at the distal end of CAF can't be detected. Multiplanar TEE can accurately display the origin, course, and drainage site of CAF, but it also has some limitations. Chung PC believes that TEE is more effective and valuable than other examination methods in the diagnosis and intra-operative monitoring of CAF (Figure 8-27).

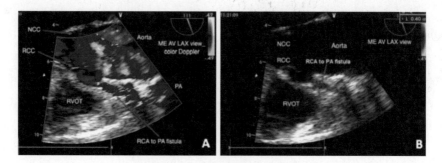

Figure 8-27   TEE of RCA-PA fistula.

(1) The RCA fistula draining into RV or RA: The dilated RCA can be observed on the conventional LV long axis section and apical five chamber section. The dilated vessels can be traced along RV wall to the lower part of the tricuspid annulus (atrioventricular groove). When scanning from the long axis to short axis of LV, the dilated RCA fistula and its course can be clearly displayed. Some patients may form giant AN within the course of CAF. The fistula orifice draining into RV is mostly located in the right atrioventricular groove, RV cone, or diaphragmatic surface. The fistula draining into RA is generally located in the anterior wall, posterior wall of RA, or the opening of SVC. Therefore, CDFI can detect the multicolored high-speed blood flow signals in the cardiac cavity where the fistula is located. The beginning of the blood flow bundle is the origin of CAF, and its width is the size of the fistula.

Eldeib M reported a new diagnostic approach to identifying CAF using an intracoronary injection of SonoVue contrast agent (Figure 8-28).

(2) LCA fistula draining into RV or RA: This type of CAF is relatively rare, and not easy to find the dilated LCA and its course in the long axis section of LV, while the dilated LCA is usually clearly seen in the short axis section and the apical five chamber section. Its dilation degree is less significant than that of RCA fistula, and CAF is generally long, tortuous, and complex. It is necessary to display various abnormal blood flow signals by CDFI, such as string-like changes (Figure 8-29).

(3) CAF draining into PA: Most of the involved coronary arteries drain

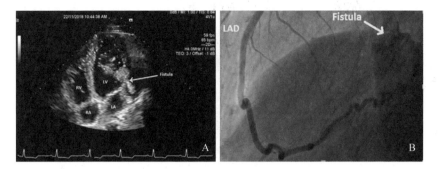

Figure 8-28 A: Apical 4 chamber view demonstrated the contrast coming from the posterior mitral annulus at LV base; B: ICA showed long LAD, continuing beyond the cardiac apex, running the full course of LCX ends by fistula to the cardiac chamber.

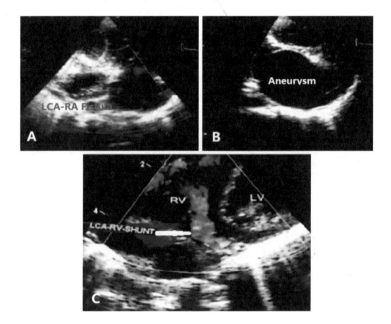

Figure 8-29 A & B: Echo of LCA-RA fistula with giant AN; C: LCA-RV fistula.

into PA. The fistula lumen is small and is not easy to be detected by two-dimensional Echo. Generally, on the long axis section of PA at the left edge of the sternum, CDFI shows the fire-like abnormal blood flow bundle in PA. On the short axis section of the large artery, CDFI also display whether the coronary artery is widened and whether there are abnormal branches. Lim

WH reported a case of RCA-PA fistula found by routine Echo (Figure 8-30).

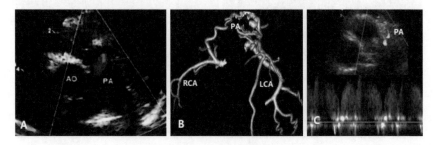

Figure 8-30 Echo (A & C) and CTA image (B) of LCA-PA fistula and RCA-PA fistula.

(4) CAF draining into the left heart system: Such patients are rare, and relevant literature points out that those who drain into LV are easy to be misdiagnosed. Because LV and aortic pressure in the systolic period are the same and there is no shunt between them, the blood flow signal in the systolic period is subtle. Only when the aortic pressure is greater than LV pressure in the diastolic period, does abnormal blood flow occur. Jung C also reported a rare CAF found by routine Echo (Figure 8-31).

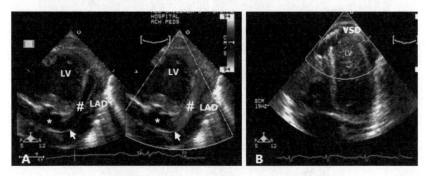

Figure 8-31 Echo of LAD-LV fistula (A) with VSD (B).

Wang F reported 2 cases of RCA fistula by two-dimensional Echo and CDFI in 1990. Two patients were initially diagnosed with ruptured sinus of Valsalva aneurysm, PDA, and aortic valve disease, and one of them was confirmed as RCA fistula by ICA and surgery. The Echo features of RCA fistula were as followings: (a) RCA fistula was abnormally large (1.2–1.5 cm in diameter); (b) There was a ring-like structure in the right atrioventricular sulcus; (c) Continuous turbulence can be detected in RCA fistula and at its entrance. The authors believe that when continuous murmurs are heard in the anterior area of the heart, especially when the pressure difference is not significant, and the clinical situation is not in accordance with PDA, VSD and aortic regurgitation or sinus aneurysm, Echo and ICA should be performed in time.

Yang Q retrospectively analyzed 11 cases of adult CAF confirmed by ICA. The authors believe that Echo is the first choice for the examination of CAF and has important clinical application value in the selection of treatment schemes and the evaluation of intra-operative and post-operative efficacy

Xiao Z and other authors think that CAF can be diagnosed by CDFI combined with spectral Doppler Echo (Figure 8-32). Gul A reported a case of double coronary arteries-LV fistula diagnosed prenatally and confirmed by surgery after delivery (Figure 8-33).

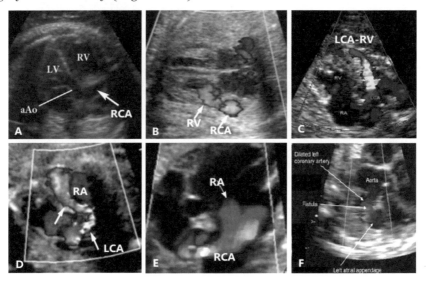

Figure 8-32　A: RCA-RV fistula; B: RCA-RV fistula; C: LCA-RV fistula; D: LCA-RA fistula; E: RCA-RA fistula; F: LCA-LA fistula.

Cotton JL reported a case of LCA-RV fistula with progression to spontaneous closure. A 23-year-old woman was referred for fetal Echo at 30 weeks because of abnormal Echo screening at 28 weeks that revealed mildly

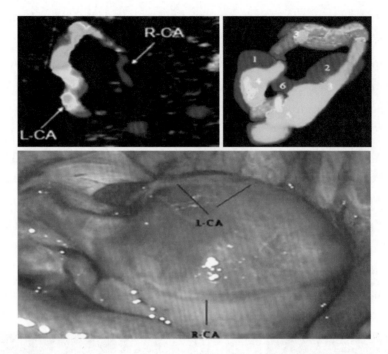

Figure 8-33   Echo and operative field of double coronary arteries-LV fistula.

dilated RV. On the fetal Echo, the heart had a normal axis with intact cardiac segment connections; RA and RV enlargement was seen with normal biventricular function; A shunt was noted from the interventricular septum into RV by CDFI, and it was determined to be diastolic by the timing of RV inflow and outflow. A diagnosis of LAD-RV fistula was made, and the patient was delivered by the caesarian section at 34 weeks because of prolonged rupture of membranes. The birth weight was 1,760 g. The postnatal Echo confirmed the prenatal diagnosis. There was dilated LAD with the prominent diastolic flow into RV. The patient did not show any signs of CHF and was treated conservatively with observation. After discharge, the patient was lost to follow-up until 1 year of age. At that visit, no cardiac murmur was appreciated, and Echo revealed no evidence of fistula patency (Figure 8-34).

Deng H retrospectively analyzed the results of TTE in 43 cases of congenital CAF and compared them with the surgical pathological results. The Echo manifestations of CAF are widening of the initial segment of the

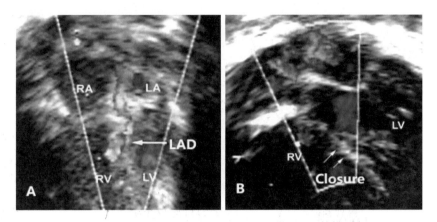

Figure 8-34   A: Postnatal apical 4-chamber view demonstrated length of fistula from LAD draining into RV; B: Apical 4-chamber view at 1 year of age, no flow through the fistula (arrows) could be documented by color flow scanning.

coronary artery, tortuous expansion of the fistula and drainage into the heart cavity or large vessel, abnormal blood flow signals at the fistula orifice, etc. The authors believe that TTE can be the first choice for noninvasive diagnosis of congenital CAF. Combining ICA for small and multiple fistulas is still recommended (Figure 8-35).

Liu Q retrospectively analyzed 11 children with CAF to find the image characteristics and regularities of CAF. The results showed that all children were correctly diagnosed by CDE. CDE of CAF has obvious image characteristics: a. CDFI shows abnormal blood flow signals in the fistula orifice of the cardiac cavity or PA; b. The involved coronary artery was obviously dilated; c. RCA-right heart system fistulas are common; d. When the fistula enters RA, RV, LA, and PA, it is a two-phase continuous turbulence spectrum, and when the fistula enters LV, it is a diastolic turbulence spectrum. The authors believe that CDE has great application value in diagnosing CAF (Figure 8-36).

When an abnormal blood flow signal in the cardiac cavity is found by Echo and suspected to be CAF, it should be distinguished from the following diseases:

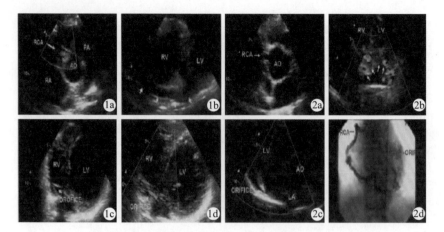

Figure 8-35 Echo of RCA-RV/LV fistula. 1a-1d: RCA-RV fistula. 1a: RCA widened and its blood flow accelerated (arrow); 1b: RCA ran in the posterior atrioventricular groove (arrow); 1c: Fistula dilatation, opening in RV; 1d: Blood flow turbulence signal at the fistula. 2a-2d: RCA-LV fistula. 2a: Dilatation of RCA; 2b: Turbulence signal in tortuous fistula (arrow); 2c: Fistula blood flow in the posterior inferior wall of LV; 2d: ICA showed RCA-LV fistula.

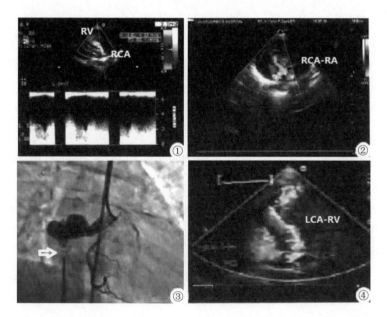

Figure 8-36 Echo of CCF. ① RCA-RV fistula; ② RCA-RA fistula; ③ Interventional closure of RCA-RA fistula; ④ LCA-LV fistula.

a. VSD (especially muscular VSD): The abnormal blood flow signal is the transseptal flow crossing the ventricular septum, which is clear in systole. But in CAF patients, we can observe the non-transseptal and diastolis signal originating from the atrioventricular wall;

b. Aortic valve regurgitation (AVR): AVR originates from the valvular edge and blood flow singal appears in the systole, while CAF originates from the atrioventricular wall or the ventricular wall near the valve root, which is mostly continuous biphasic flow in the diastole;

c. Aorticopulmonary septal defect: This disease can be seen at the level of PA, and the interval between the aorta and PA is missing to varying degrees. The local blood flow shows a turbulent color spectrum, while the septum between the aorta and PA of CAF is complete;

d. Coronary sinus dilatation: It is easy to misdiagnose. The low-speed venous flow spectrum is in CS, while the high-speed turbulent signal is in the dilated CAF;

e. Kawasaki disease: Only local dilation of the coronary artery is shown, but no abnormal blood flow signal is found in the cardiac cavity or PA.

Some scholars put forward the Echo findings for diagnosing CAF:

a. The diameter of the involved coronary artery was significantly enlarged.

b. Begin from the origin of the coronary artery and constantly change the angle and orientation of the probe to track the coronary artery to the fistula.

c. Color and spectral Doppler can detect the high-speed turbulence signal at the fistula. Except for the diastolic turbulence when the fistula enters LV, the rest are systolic and diastolic continuous turbulence. It may be accompanied by ventricular and aortic dilatation with insufficiency of the aortic valve.

Section IV   CT and MR

Magnetic resonance (MR) and MDCT or CTA can be used as critical auxiliary means of angiography. MR multiplanar reconstruction can clearly show the course and the inflow or outflow of abnormal blood vessels (Figures 8-37, 8-38); cardiovascular MDCT or CTA images can clearly display the distal and collateral vessels of the coronary artery, and can obtain 3-D images of the coronary artery in a short time (Figures 8-39, 8-40). MDCT and CTA can not only clearly show the anatomical relationship between CAF and adjacent tissues, but also the drainage site (Figures 8-41, 8-42, and 8-43).

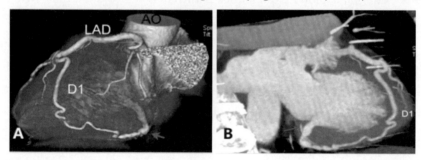

Figure 8-37 A 67-year-old male with no symptoms. Volume rendering and maximum intensity projection images showed dilated and tortuous fistula between first diagonal artery (D1) and RV. The drainage site of CAF was shown clearly (arrow).

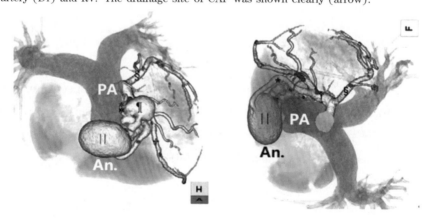

Figure 8-38   CT images before the procedure showed CAPF and 2 giant AN

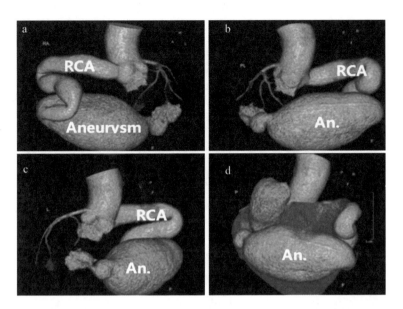

Figure 8-39   Coronary CTA. Serpentine RCA and the giant saccular AN located in the distal portions of RCA, the diffusely dilated fistula drained into LV. a: left-anterior oblique view; b: right-posterior oblique view; c: posteroanterior view; d: The giant saccular AN (up to 6.1 cm) surrounded RV.

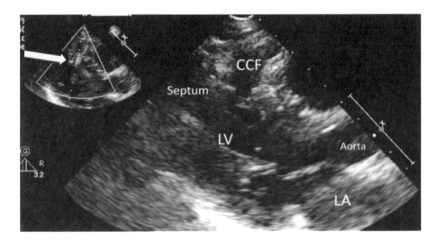

Figure 8-40   Parasternal long-axis view showed CCF with abnormal diastolic color flow signal (arrow) to LV.

CTA can well demonstrate the origins and terminations, the course, classification, and lesions of peripheral cardiac microvessel of CAF, and play

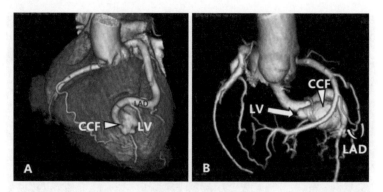

Figure 8-41 3-D CT showed the LV side (arrow) and LAD (curved arrow) of CCF (arrowhead).

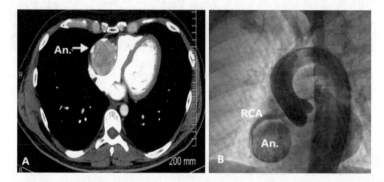

Figure 8-42 A: Contrast-enhanced CT showed the 5 cm × 5 cm × 5 cm right-sided cardiac mass (arrow); B: ICA of the aortic root showed RCA aneurysm, which supplied the posterior descending coronary artery and the posterolateral branch.

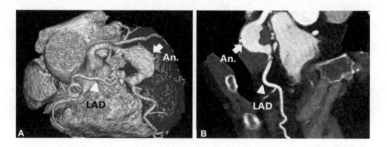

Figure 8-43 MDCT of the coronary artery. A: Reconstructed image showed saccular AN (arrow) of LAD with fistula (arrowhead) from the conus artery to PA; B: LAD (arrowhead) and aneurysmal sac (arrow).

an essential role in the clinical diagnosis, treatment planning, and post-operative evaluation of CAF (Figures 8-44, 8-45, 8-46, 8-47, 8-48, and 8-49).

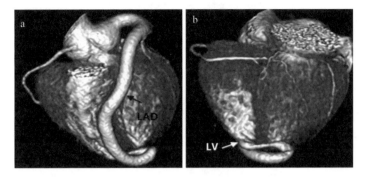

Figure 8-44   A 4-year-old girl presented with progressive dyspnea. CTA images demonstrated a short fistula tract of end-artery type. Dilated LAD (black arrow in a) terminates into LV (white arrow in b).

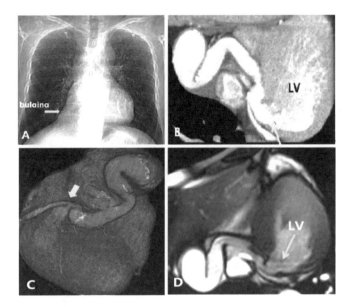

Figure 8-45   A 42-year-old male with aneurysmal CCF. A: Cardiac bulging to the right; B & D: CT and MR indicated the draining of CCF into LV base with a flow jet (yellow arrow); C: The tortuous course followed along the posterior atrioventricular groove before draining into LV (short yellow arrow).

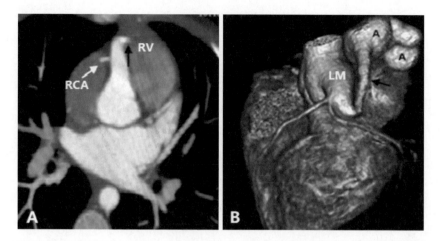

Figure 8-46 A: A 4-year-old girl. CTA image demonstrated a short fistula tract. The fistula originates from the proximal RCA and terminates into RV (black arrow). The normal RCA distal to the fistula was patent (white arrow); B: A 1-year-old boy. CTA image demonstrated fistula (black arrow) originating from LM associated with multiple AN.

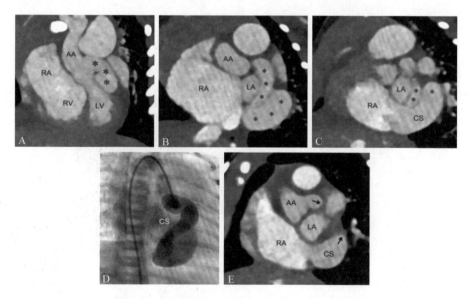

Figure 8-47 Coronary artery-CS fistula. A-C: CT images showed the severely dilated LCX (asterisks) anomalously draining into the dilated CS in a 3-day-old girl; D: ICA performed on the same day confirming the diagnosis of CCF fistula; E: Follow-up CT image performed one month after surgical ligation of the fistula showed stumps (arrows) of LCX and CS.

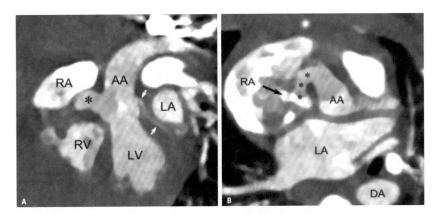

Figure 8-48   CCF between RCA and RA in an 11-day-old boy. A: CT image showed the severely dilated origin and proximal portion of RCA (asterisk). LCA (white arrows) was normal in size; B: CT image revealed the fistulous connection (arrow) between the dilated proximal RCA (asterisks) and RA.

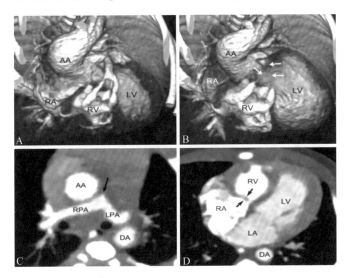

Figure 8-49. Ventriculo-coronary arterial connections in a 1-day-old girl with pulmonary atresia, an intact ventricular septum, and hypoplastic tricuspid valve. CT images obtained at the end-systolic (A) and end-diastolic (B) phases showed the severely dilated LAD and the mildly dilated RCA connected to the hypoplastic RV at multiple sites. Notably, diastolic flow to LAD was significantly compromised (arrows), which may contribute to myocardial ischemia; C: CT image demonstrated pulmonary atresia (arrow) with confluent central branch pulmonary arteries; D: CT image showed the hypoplastic tricuspid valve (arrows), the hypoplastic RV, and the intact ventricular septum.

CTA combined with 3-D visualization reconstruction technology can intuitively and accurately display the morphologic features of CAF, and can be used as the first choice for the diagnosis of CAF (Figure 8-50).

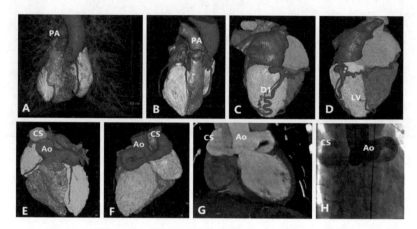

Figure 8-50 A: Coronary-PA fistula could be seen. The origin artery was the right conus branch, and the fistula was tortuous; B: The fistula located on the atrial side of PA; C & D: The distal end of the first diagonal branch was extended and tortuous to form a main fistula, which entered LV and was a single fistula; E-H: LM was tortuous and extended, running between aorta and LA, and fistula into SVC.

Many case reports and reviews showed that CTA could clearly demonstrate the anatomy of the coronary artery, the site of the closure device and the presence or absence of residual shunt, which is valuable in post-operative follow-up (Figures 8-51, 8-52 and 8-53).

Ouchi K observed a 0.91% prevalence of CAF determined with cardiac CT, with LAD as the most common site of origin (67.7%) and the main PA as the most common site of drainage (82.3%). The incidence of AN accompanying CAF was 48.4%. The results differed from those reported based on CAG. In addition, abnormal flow in CDFI might suggest that CAF was likely undetectable. Cardiac CT allows noninvasive and comprehensive assessment of CAF and is required to establish the cause of continuous murmur that is not identified with TTE (Figures 8-54, 8-55).

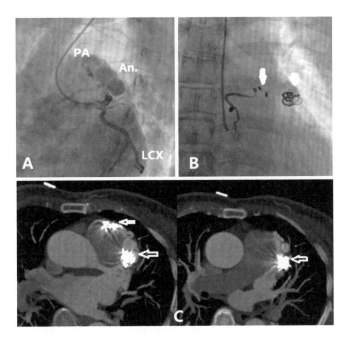

Figure 8-51   One year after TCC (arrows), the patients with multiple CAPF underwent coronary CTA. The fistula was basically blocked completely, without contrast agent filling in the tumor-like expansion, and there were still small fistulas connected to PA.

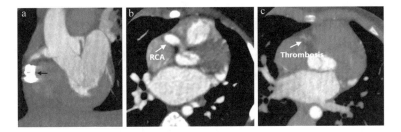

Figure 8-52   CTA after 8 months of TCC (2-year-old boy). a: An oblique sagittal section demonstrated closure devices of RCA-RV fistula (black arrow); b & c: CT images demonstrated patent RCA before TCC (b) and coronary thrombosis after TCC (white arrow in c).

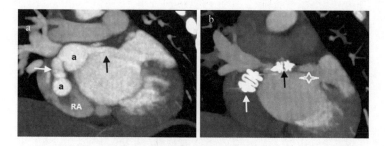

Figure 8-53   CTA after 6 months of TCC (4-year-old boy). CTA demonstrated partial fistula thrombosis after TCC. a: LM-RA fistula (black arrow) contained 2 AN. The fistula tract between 2 AN was relatively small (white arrow); b: A fistula tract (asterisk) proximal to device closure (arrows) was still patented.

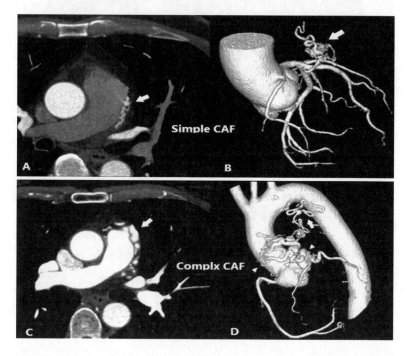

Figure 8-54   CT image of simple CAF in a 54-year-old man (A & B) and complex CAF in a 57-year-old woman (C & D). Axial (A) and volume-rendered images (B) showed a single fistulous connection from the conus branch of LAD into the main PA (arrow). Axial (C) and volume-rendered images (D) showed several prominent and separate (arrowhead) fistulous connections from LAD, LCX, and RCA. These branches entered the main PA (arrow in C) and continued with the bronchial arteries arising from the descending thoracic aorta (arrow in D).

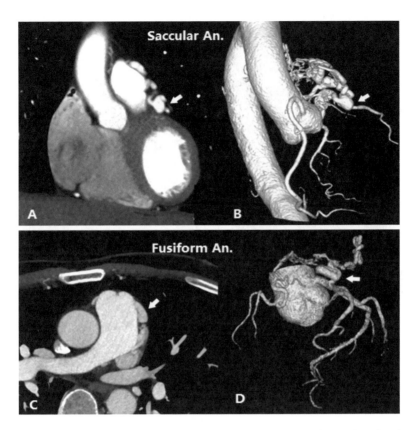

Figure 8-55 CT image of AN accompanying CAF. A & B: Coronal and volume-rendered images showed a saccular AN of the fistulous track (arrow) in a 57-year-old woman; C & D: Axial and volume-rendered images showed a fusiform AN of a tortuous fistulous track (arrow) in a 52-year-old man.

ECG-gated CTA with 3-D reconstruction can accurately assess the complex anatomy of CAF, including the site and the number of origins, drainage sites, and associated anomalies. This information is essential for therapeutic planning. Therefore, in order to aid clinicians in making appropriate clinical and therapeutic decisions, radiologists should be fully aware of the critical role of CTA in evaluating CAF (Figures 8-56, 8-57, 8-58, 8-59, 8-60, and 8-61).

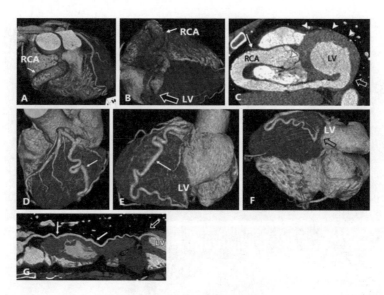

Figures 8-56 A-C: A 42-year-old man with a heart murmur. A & B: Volume-rendered CT images obtained at different levels showed a diffusely dilated RCA (white arrow) along the arterioventricular groove and draining into LV chamber (black arrow in B); C: Curved multiplanar reformatted CT image depicted a fistulous communication between the dilated RCA (white arrow) and LV chamber (black arrow). LV hypertrophy (arrowheads) was due to increased blood volume in the left cardiac chamber. D & G: CCF in a 55-year-old man. D & F: Volume-rendered CT images obtained at different levels showed a diffusely dilated obtuse marginal branch (arrow in D and E) draining into LV chamber (arrow in F). G: Curved multiplanar reformatted CT image depicted a fistulous communication between the dilated obtuse marginal branch (white arrows) and LV chamber (black arrow).

Cai R analyzed the difference between the CAPF group (380) and the CCF group (99). Among 96,037 patients, 482 (0.5%) patients (232 male and 250 female) had CAF. The PA was the most common site of drainage (380/482, 78.8%). Of the 99 CCF, coronary to LV was the most common pattern in CCF (34/482, 7.0%). Single origin was more common in CAF (n = 361, 74.9%), and multiple origins were more common in CAPF than in CCF. There were statistically significant differences in the stoma diameter (2.4 ± 1.1 mm vs. 5.4 ± 4.3 mm, $p < 0.05$), complicated with AN (85 cases [85/380] vs. 50 cases [50/99]), the size of AN (8.8 ± 5.7 mm vs. 19.1 ± 11.6 mm, $p < 0.05$), and single fistula (261 [261/380] vs. 96 [96/99], $p < 0.05$).

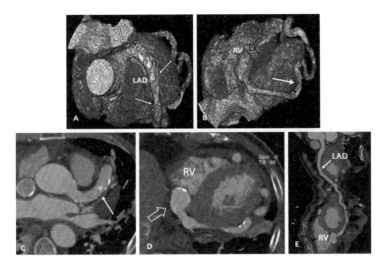

Figure 8-57　CCF in a 63-year-old man who presented with dyspnea. A & B: Volume-rendered CT images obtained at different levels showed a dilated and calcified LAD (closed arrows) coursing along the anterior and posterior interventricular grooves into RV chamber (open arrow in B), representing a left-right shunt; C & D: Axial CT images showed CCF originating from the dilated LAD (arrow in C) and draining into RV chamber (arrow in D). Note the bulbous change in the fistulous tract at the entrance to RV chamber; E: Curved multiplanar reformatted CT image showed a fistulous communication between the dilated LAD (arrow) and RV chamber.

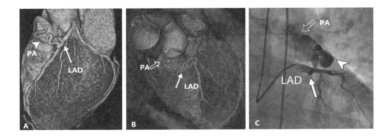

Figure 8-58　Coronary-PA fistula in a 55-year-old man with dyspnea. A-B: Volume-rendered CT images obtained at different levels showed a single prominent fistulous connection from the conus branch of LAD (solid arrow) into the main pulmonary trunk (open arrow in B); C: ICA confirmed the presence of coronary-PA fistula, with single prominent tract, originating from the proximal LAD (solid arrow) and draining into the main PA (open arrow). Note the focal aneurysmal change in the fistulous tract (arrowhead in A and C).

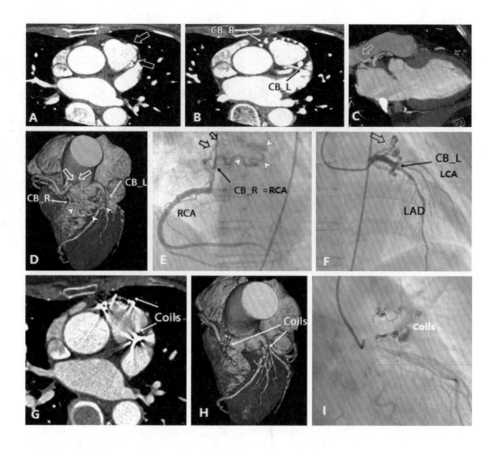

Figure 8-59   Coronary-PA fistula in a 62-year-old man who underwent TCC. A-F: CT images before TCC. A & B: Axial CT images showed multiple dilated fistulous connections and a tortuous fistulous tract arising from RCA and LAD (arrows in B) into the main PA (arrows in A); C: Two-chamber reformatted CT image showed the contrast shunt sign created as a jet of contrast material flushes into the relatively less-opacified PA (arrow); D & F: Volume-rendered CT image and ICA showed the Vieussens ring (arrowheads in D and E), composed of the conus branches of LAD and RCA (solid arrows). In this case, CAF are originated from 2 vessels: 3 mm conus branch of RCA and 3 mm conus branch of LAD. The drainage site was the main PA (open arrows), and the fistulous tract course was the pre-pulmonary trunk, anterior to RVOT. No accompanying cardiac abnormalities are seen; G & I: Axial CT image, volume-rendered CT image, and ICA after successful TCC showed no residual fistula. The fistula tract was completely obliterated, with no evidence of recanalization, persistent coronary artery dilatation, or thrombus.

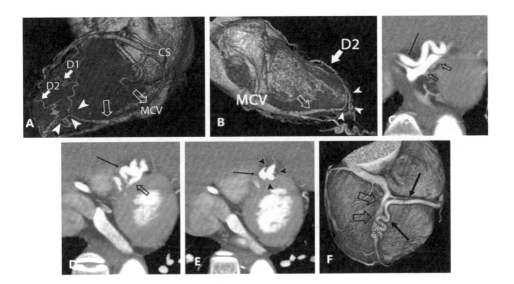

Figures 8-60   Coronary artery-cardiac vein fistula in a 57-year-old woman
with chest pain. A & B: Volume-rendered CT images obtained at different
levels showed tortuous first (D1) and second (D2) diagonal branches of LAD
(solid arrows) connected to the dilated middle cardiac vein (MCV) (open
arrows), which drained into CS. Arrowheads point to connecting points
between D1 or D2 of LAD and the middle cardiac vein; C & F: Coronary
artery-cardiac vein fistula in a 51-year-old woman with exertional dyspnea;
Serial axial CT images showed a dilated tortuous PDA from RCA (long arrow)
along the posterior interventricular groove, draining into the middle cardiac
vein (short arrows in C and E). Arrowheads point to the connecting point
between PDA and middle cardiac vein (C); F: Volume-rendered CT image also
showed the fistulous connection between the dilated tortuous PDA of RCA
(solid arrows) and the middle cardiac vein (open arrows), * indicates the
connecting point.

Most of the 380 CAPF patients received conservative treatments (350/380,
92.1%), while the 59 CCF patients (59/93, 63.4%) were treated. The main
imaging manifestations of CAF: small fistulas at the end of the main coronary
artery and branches or side branches are connected to the heart cavity or PA;
one or more small tortuous abnormally anastomotic branches of the

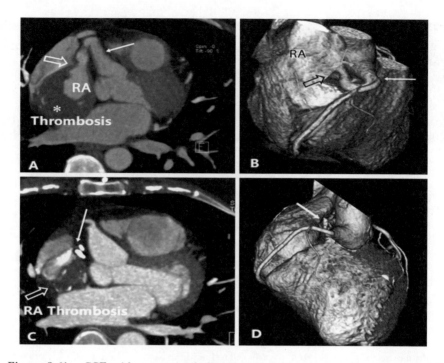

Figure 8-61　　CCF with a proximal thrombosed RCA aneurysm in a 39-year-old woman who subsequently underwent surgical ligation. A & B: Pre-procedural axial and volume-rendered CT images showed dilated RCA (solid arrow), which draining into RA (open arrow). Note the thrombus (* in A) in RA, adjacent to a dilated fistulous tract from RCA. In this case, CAF has a single fistulous tract of large diameter (1 cm). The fistulous tract passed through the right atrioventricular groove and drained into the anterior surface of RA; C & D: On post-procedural axial and volume-rendered CT images, there was no visualization of the residual fistulous tract between RCA and RA owing to successful ligation of the proximal dilated RCA. The solid arrow indicated surgical clips. The fistula tract was completely obliterated at the proximal portion, without evidence of recanalization or persistent coronary artery dilatation. However, a residual thrombosed AN was noted at the stumped portion of the fistulous tract in RA (open arrow in C).

coronary arteries; the coronary artery dilates markedly, forming AN (Figures 8-62, 8-63, 8-64, 8-65, and 8-66).

　　Some domestic scholars used more than 256 slice spiral CTA to examine and diagnose coronary-PA fistula. The authors believe that the CTA technique has various recombination methods, which can intuitively and accurately display the abnormal vascular morphology and ejection signs of

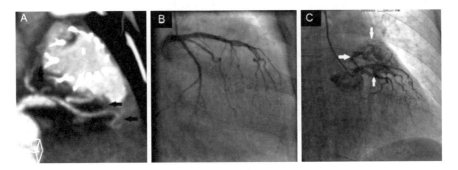

Figure 8-62   A 73-year-old woman with LCX-LA fistula after LAA occlusion. (A) MIP showed the multivessel structure (arrows) from LCX draining into LAA; (B) ICA showed that there were no abnormalities before surgery; (C) LCX leaked into LA after LAA occlusion, resulting in contrast agent concentration (arrows).

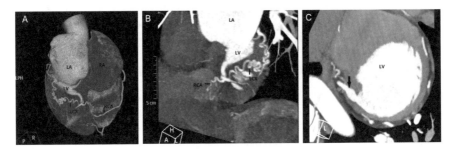

Figure 8-63   A 38-year-old woman with RCA/LCX-LV fistula. (A)(B) Volume-rendered images and MIP showed complex CCF between RCA/LCX and LV (arrows); (C) They were finally drained into LV (arrow).

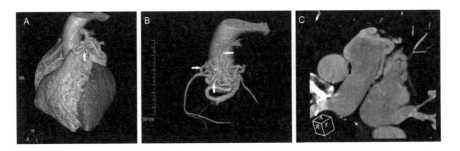

Figure 8-64   A 38-year-old man with LAD-PA fistula. Volume-rendered images and MIP showed tortuous ectatic vascular structure (arrows in A & B) from LAD draining into PA (arrow in C).

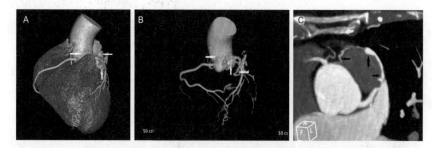

Figure 8-65 A 64-year-old woman with multiple vessels fistula into PA. Volume-rendered images and MIP showed tortuous vascular structure (arrows in A & B) from LAD and RCA draining into PA (arrows in C).

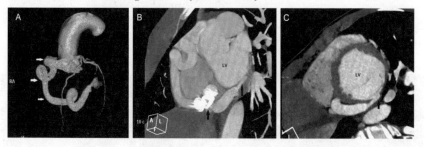

Figure 8-66 A 15-year-old man with RCA-LV fistula. Volume-rendered images and MIP showed ectatic vascular structure (arrow in A) from the RCA draining into LV; MIP showed the fistula tract was still existed after interventional treatment with an asymmetrical umbrella blocker through RV (black arrows in B & C).

CAF. It can directly observe the hairball or sieve distribution of the abnormal vascular masses, the formation of AN, and mild to moderate stenosis. CTA can clearly understand the anatomical structure of CAF and help doctors to diagnose complex CAF (Figure 8-67).

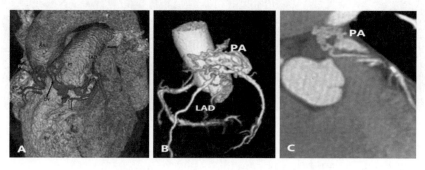

Figure 8-67 CT images of LAD-PA fistula.

Park JH reported the incidence of CAF in South Korea and believed that CT examination was of great value in diagnosing CAF. Likewise, early SA. and others believed that CT examination could determine the direction and location of the fistula (Figures 8-68, 8-69, 8-70, 8-71, and 8-72).

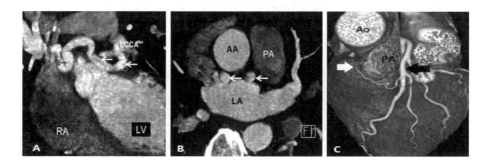

Figure 8-68   A: LCA-RA fistula; B: Coronary-LA fistula; C: LAD-PA fistula.

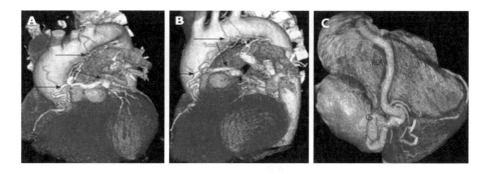

Figure 8-69   A & B: The rave and complex CAF. Artery-artery fistula emanating from RCA, RCA-PA fistula; C: RCA-CS fistula.

Cheng Z and others retrospectively analyzed the clinical findings and imaging data of children with CAF. All children underwent low-dose prospective ECG-gated MDCT angiography. The accuracy of CT diagnosis of CAF was calculated based on surgery or traditional angiography results. The results showed that the CT images of all children were diagnosable with a subjective score of (2.6 ±0.7) and a good consistency between the 2 physicians. Therefore the authors believe low-dose DSCT angiography can be

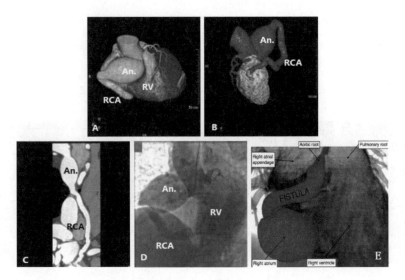

Figure 8-70   A-D: CT images and angiogram of RCA-RV fistula;
E: CT showed RCA-RA fistula.

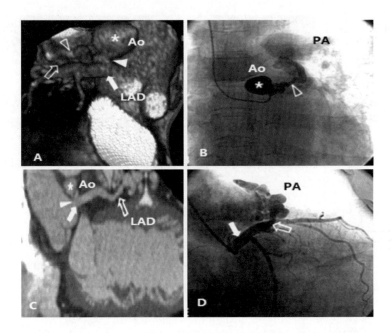

Figure 8-71   CT images (A, C) and angiograms (B, D) of ascending aorta and
LAD-PA fistula. There were 2 fistulas in PA, one of which originated from the
ascending aorta and the other branch originated from LAD.

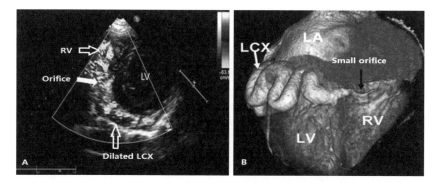

Figure 8-72   Echo and CT image of LCX-RV fistula.

used as an accurate and reliable noninvasive imaging method for diagnosing CAF in children (Figure 8-73).

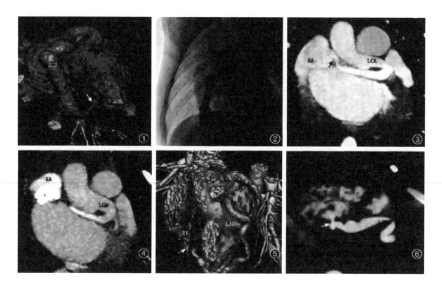

Figure 8-73   CT images of CAF in children. ①② RCA-RV fistula in a 1-year-old female child; ③④ LCA-RA fistula in a 9-month-old male child; ⑤⑥ LAD-RV fistula in a 3-year-old male child.

Cao H reconstructed the patient-specific 3-D CAF model of a 38-year-old male patient based on CT images and then employed computational fluid dynamics (CFD) to quantify changes in hemodynamic parameters before and after fistula closure, aiming to estimate the effectiveness of improving blood-stealing and determine whether there are any geometrical or hemodynamic factors. This study will help to understand the related factors leading to thrombosis after fistula closure, identify the key parameters for predictions of clinical outcomes, and assist in the decision-making of potential anticoagulant treatments (Figures 8-74, 8-75, and 8-76).

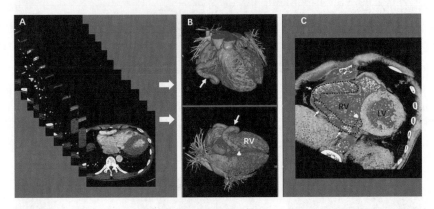

Figure 8-74 A: Original thin-slice CT image stacks used for 3-D reconstruction; B: Volume rendered technique showed marked dilated RCA (white arrows); C: Volume rendered technique demonstrated RCA (white arrows) was connected to RV. Note the orifice of coronary-RV fistula (white arrowhead).

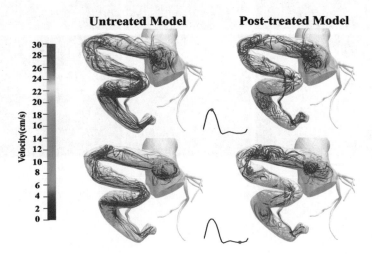

Figure 8-75 Streamlines in the dilated RCA for all models at the peak systole and diastole. The velocity magnitudes were differentiated by using a color bar.

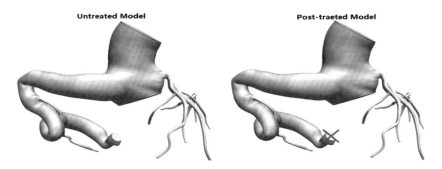

Figure 8-76   3-D reconstructed models based on CT images. The orifice of CAF was patent before TCC (untreated model), while it was occluded in post-treated model.

Uchida T showed intra-operative fluorescence-guided images for CAF (Figures 8-77, 8-78). Mitamura K presented a case of giant CAF with abnormal findings on 123 I-MIBG scintigraphy (Figures 8-79, 8-80).

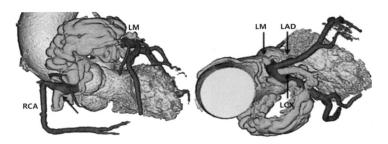

Figure 8-77   CT showed CAF to PA originating from RCA, LM and LCX (arrows).

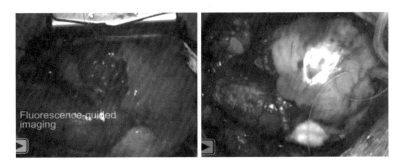

Figure 8-78   After injection of Indocyanine green, intra-operative fluorescence image using a photodynamic eye clearly demonstrated fistulous vessels. No abnormal vessels were visualized after ligation and resection of fistulous vessels.

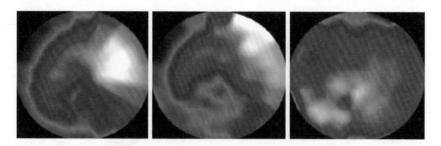

Figure 8-79　123 I-MIBG polar map. On both early and late phase images, decreased accumulation was depicted in the apical to basal inferior wall. Diffuse high washout especially in the apical to basal inferior wall was observed.

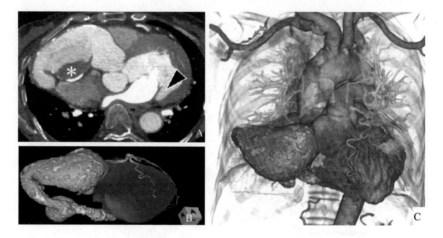

Figure 8-80　A: CTA images demonstrated tortuous RCA with marked diffuse aneurysmal dilation draining into the basal inferolateral wall of LV (black arrowhead) and also showed a filling defect at the proximal region of the RCA (∗); B: Hybrid 123 I-MIBG SPECT image. A reduced accumulation in the inferior wall was located in RCA territory; C: CT image showed giant RCA at the right lower lung field.

Salavitabar A used multimodality imaging to demonstrate an unusual embryologic remnant (Figures 8-81, 8-82). Guglielmo M showed multimodality images of LCX-RA fistula associated with giant AN (Figure 8-83).

Miura S considered through the novel case that the myocardial ischemia before surgery was likely due to the coronary steal phenomenon. Worsened ischemia after surgery was likely due to thrombotic occlusion of RCA aneurysm. Overall, 13 N-ammonia PET/CT can help assess the functional

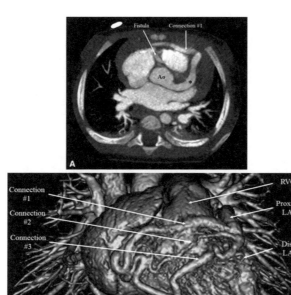

Figure 8-81   A: CTA showed severely dilated LM and LAD (∗) with no evidence of RCA ostium, intercoronary ' Connection #1' coursing anteriorly, and the fistula coursing toward RV outflow tract in an oblique axial plane; B: 3-D volume-rendered CTA.

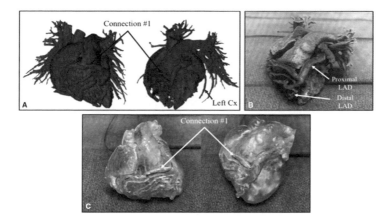

Figure 8-82   A: 3-D virtual model from the anteroposterior (left) and lateral (right) views; B: 3D-printed model with LAD as labeled; C: 3D-printed model with coronary arteries and inter-coronary connections hollowed out. A wire was seen coursing from the ostium of LM, through LAD, and into intercoronary "Connection #1".

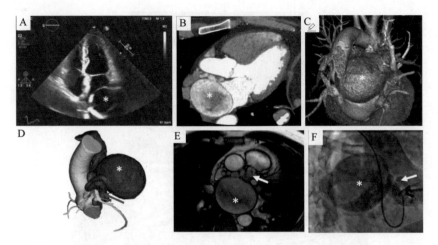

Figure 8-83 A 46-year-old man with a history of palpitation and 24-h Holter monitoring demonstrated only mild supraventricular ectopic beats, and TTE showed a large anechoic chamber with slow flow inside, compressing LA (A). CTA showed proximal LCX giving rise to dilated and tortuous CAF draining into giant AN compressing LA; AN itself drained into a kinked vessel coursing posteriorly to aorta and PA, winding laterally around SVC and eventually terminating into RA (B-D). The mid and distal LCX had normal calibre. No significant CAD was noted. CMR confirmed the presence of CAF, demonstrated normal biventricular cavity size and systolic function, normal biatrial size, and normal pulmonary to systemic flow ratio, and ruled out AN thrombosis (E). A coronary angiogram was also performed (F).

status and quantify coronary blood flow in patients with CAA. A 60-year-old woman with a known RCA-CS fistula presented with 2-month history of dyspnea, chest tightness on exertion and persistent atrial tachycardia. Chest X-ray revealed biventricular dilation, which had not been seen 7 years ago. TTE showed normal LV ejection fraction with no wall motion abnormalities, enlargement of all 4 chambers, and left-right shunt with Qp/Qs of 1.3. TEE demonstrated dilated and tortuous RCA, CAF between RCA and dilated CS, and stenosis of CS ostium oppressed by RCA (Figure 8-84). CTA confirmed the Echo findings: significantly dilated and tortuous RCA and single RCA-CS fistula. Additionally, the epicardial collateral vessel was visualized from LAD to RCA (Figure 8-85). 13 N-ammonia PET/CT during Adenosine triphosphate (ATP)-induced coronary hyperemia revealed a reversible perfusion

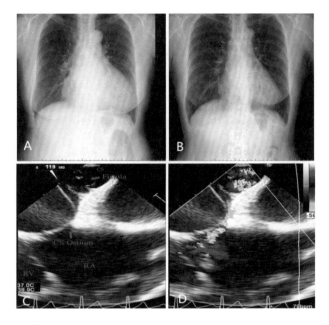

Figure 8-84   A-B: Chest X-ray revealed cardiac enlargement (cardiothoracic ratio 69%) compared with the 49% (7 years ago); C & D: Two-dimensional TEE demonstrated the massively dilated RCA and aneurysmally dilated CS. A turbulent color flow from RCA into the proximal CS was identified as a single fistula by CDFI.

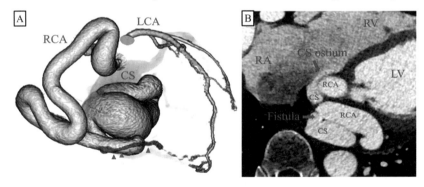

Figure 8-85   A: CTA demonstrated extremely enlarged RCA in full length with apparent aneurysmal dilatation in the terminal RCA, enormously enlarged CS in the proximal portion, and normal LCA. At maximal dilation, RCA was 36 mm and CS was 24 mm, highlighting that no epicardial branch from RCA was observed throughout the entire RCA. Instead, an epicardial collateral vessel was visualized from the distal LAD to the distal RCA (red arrowheads); B: Axial-enhanced CTA clearly depicted fistula between the terminal RCA and proximal CS with distinct visualization of the narrow CS ostium compressed by the distal RCA.

abnormality in the inferior and inferolateral regions of LV (Figure 8-86).

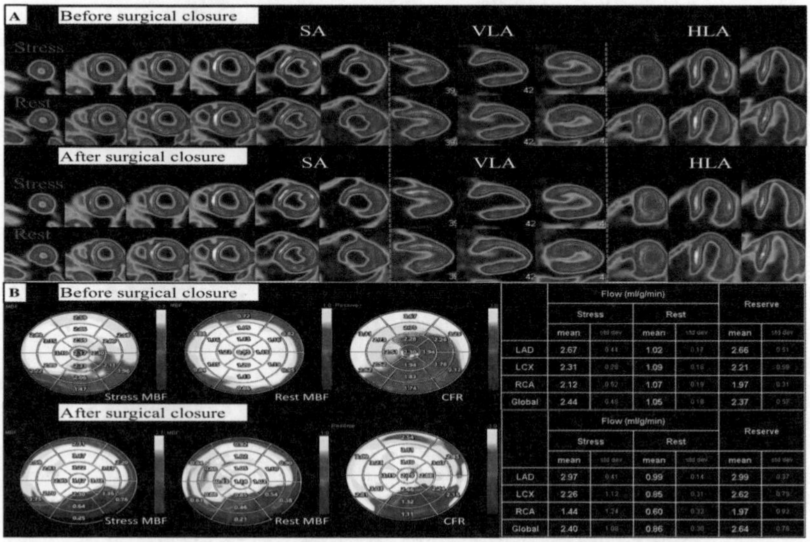

Figure 8-86 13 N-ammonia SPECT/MPI demonstrated the pre-operative reversible myocardial ischemia on the posterior walls that was significantly expanded post-operatively concerning the location and extent throughout RCA-supplied territory (A). ATP-induced stress/rest imaging was performed to quantify myocardial blood flow (MBF), myocardial perfusion, and CFR (B). Post-operatively, rest and stress MBF for RCA showed a significant decline with a substantial drop in CFR over RCA territory, suggesting severe myocardial ischemia potentially provoked by the enhanced turbulence flow effect.

The coronary flow reserve ratio (CFR) was decreased in RCA territory. The patient underwent surgical ligation of the fistula under CPB without grafting the distal RCA because of the small vessel size. PET/CT repeated 16 days after surgery, demonstrated a significant reduction in stress/rest myocardial blood flow and CFR in RCA territory with a larger area of ischemia in the affected area. For pre- and post-operative PET examinations, ECG was done at baseline and during stress with ATP infusion. Although frequent atrial arrhythmia and symptomatic hypotension complicated the post-operative course, the patient was discharged 31 days after surgery, and the 5-month post-operative follow-up was uneventful.

Lee SK evaluated the hemodynamic characteristics of CAPF using thallium-201 (Tl-201) SPECT. Tl-201 myocardial perfusion SPECT might be useful for determining hemodynamic status and risk stratification in patients with CAPF (Figure 8-87).

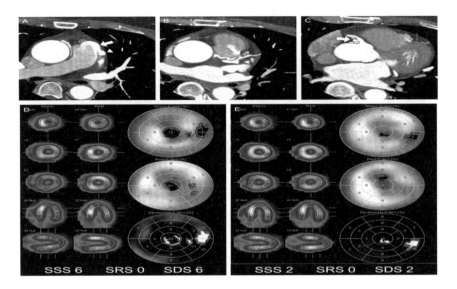

Figure 8-87　A 52-year-old woman with CAPF who underwent surgical ligation. A: Axial CTA images showed tortuous and dilated vessels around the main PA and a high-density jet flow, which directly inserted into PA (arrow). This vascular connection passed from the left side of the main PA and forms aneurysmal dilatation (arrowhead) before it entered PA; B & C: These vessels originated from 2 different vessels: from the proximal LAD (arrow in B) and from the proximal RCA (arrow in C); D: Stress and rest polar maps showed perfusion abnormality with moderate reversible ischemia; E: After surgical ligation, subsequent SPECT showed the decreased extent of the perfusion abnormality.

Junco Vicente A reported the case of a 74-year-old woman with long-standing hypertension and diabetes mellitus who underwent ICA due to oppressive chest pain on exertion. No significant obstructive lesions were detected, but LCX-dependent fistula was found (Figure 8-88).

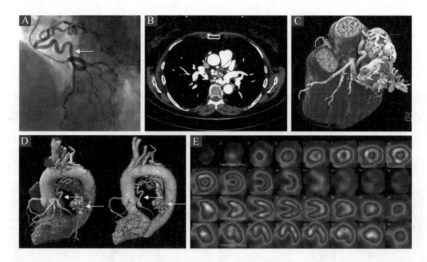

Figure 8-88   A: Angiogram showed the fistulous channel originating from LCX (arrow); B: Axial CTA showed tortuous coronary fistula (arrow); C: 3-D reconstruction of CTA; D: 3-D reconstruction of CTA showed the long fistulous duct to the bronchial arteries (arrows); E: SPECT showed normal perfusion at stress.

Section V   ICA

ICA (including CTA) is the gold standard for diagnosing CAF and is the premise of interventional therapy (Figure 8-89). It is difficult for angiography to show the abnormal tortuous vessels in one sequence clearly, and the relationship between CAF and other cardiac structures, as well as the origin and course of CAF are not well displayed.

Main signs of angiography (Figures 8-90, 8-91, 8-92, and 8-93):

(1) Most of the involved coronary arteries showed tortuous and tumor-like expansion to form fusiform or saccular AN. One fistula usually connects with the cardiac cavity or large blood vessels, and a few can see two or more multiple fistulas.

(2) In some CAF, the coronary arteries, especially the branches, are not dilated or slightly tortuous, and the terminals are connected to the cardiac cavity by multiple microvascular networks.

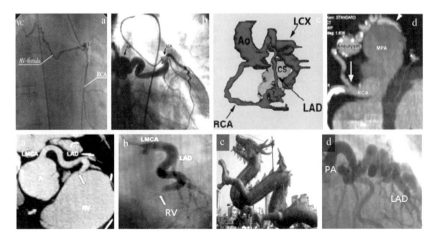

Figure 8-89 Angiogram and CT images of CAF. The top row—a: RCA-SVC fistula; b: LCA-RA fistula; c: RCA/LCX-CS fistula; d: RCA-PA fistula. The next row—a-b: LAD-RV fistula; c-d: LAD-PA fistula similar to Asian Dragon.

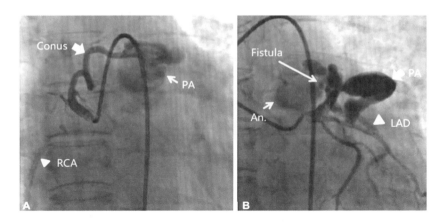

Figure 8-90 Coronary angiogram of CAF. A: RCA (arrowhead) and fistula (arrow) from the conus artery to PA (short thin arrow); B: LAD (arrowhead), aneurysmal sac (arrow), fistula (long thin arrow) from proximal LAD to PA (short thin arrow).

Fistulas arise from the right or left coronary arteries, and 90% of cases drain into PA, RV, or RA in order of decreasing frequency. Typically, young patients are asymptomatic, but supraventricular arrhythmia can be seen with progressive dilation of the intracardiac chambers. Angina can occur as the

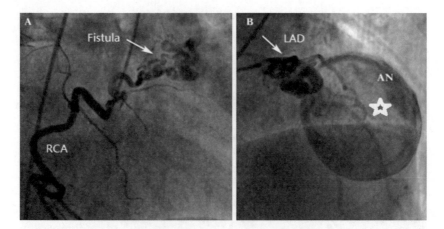

Figure 8-91   Digital subtraction coronary angiogram of CAF and AN. A: The fistulous vessels arising from the proximal RCA; B: Huge AN arising from the fistula fed by LAD, with no visible efferent vessels.

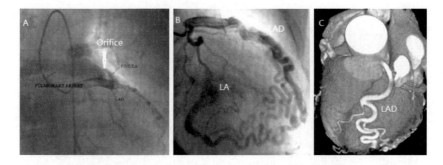

Figure 8-92   A: LAD-PA fistula; B & C: LAD-LA fistula.

fistula creates a coronary steal by diverting blood away from the myocardium. Most fistulas are associated with a small shunt; hence, the murmur is often less than grade 3/6 in the precordial area. Unless the shunt is large, the ECG is normal, as is the chest X-ray. Echo, especially the TEE, may be able to delineate the anomaly, but ICA is diagnostic. Echo studies usually suggest the site and type of fistulas. A tiny CAF to the PA, which produces no symptoms, can be detected only incidentally by an Echo study. CMR and CTA are promising additional noninvasive imaging techniques to provide detailed coronary anatomy. However, cardiac catheterization with selective ICA remains the primary modality used to define the coronary

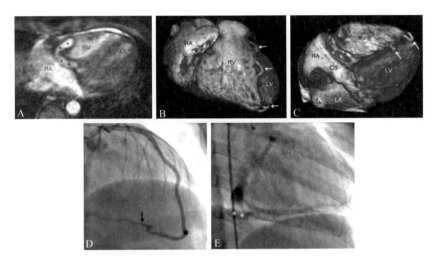

Figure 8-93   Coronary artery-middle cardiac vein fistula. A: Axial coronary MR angiographic image showed a fusiform enlarged vascular space (asterisks) at the basal portion of RV in a 2-year-old boy; B & C: Cardiac volume-rendered CT images performed 3 years later showed the mildly dilated LAD (arrows). However, the enlarged vascular space (asterisks) detected on MR was barely seen; D & E: ICA images performed 4 years later demonstrated the abnormal connection (arrow) between LAD and the middle cardiac vein, delayed opacification of the enlarged vascular space (asterisks).

anatomy, fistula size, origin and drainage site, and presence of any stenosis; it can also be used to perform a hemodynamic evaluation (Figures 8-94, 8-95, 8-96, 8-97, and 8-98).

Lin L reviewed the coronary angiographic data of 2,024 patients and confirmed 42 cases of various congenital CAA: 9 cases with the abnormal coronary origin; 33 cases of congenital CAF, including 24 cases of CAPF. Nine cases were confirmed by operation, and 2 cases of CAPF were treated by interventional embolization. Shen D also analyzed the ICA data of 1,520 adult patients retrospectively, analyzed the imaging data of 58 (3.82%) patients with CAA, and classified them according to their anatomical characteristics. Twenty-six cases (1.71%) had abnormal origin and distribution of coronary artery, and 11 cases with abnormal coronary termination were CAF, with an incidence of 0.72%.

Sasi V suggested that the coronary blood flow reserve index be used as a

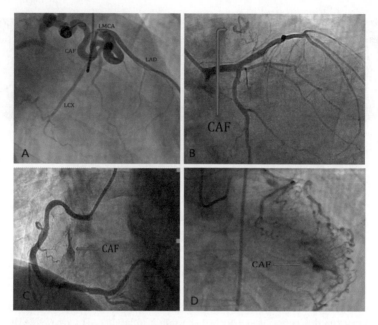

Figure 8-94 ICA images of various CAF. A: LM-RA fistula; B: LAD-PA fistula; C: RCA-RA fistula; D: LCX-LV fistula.

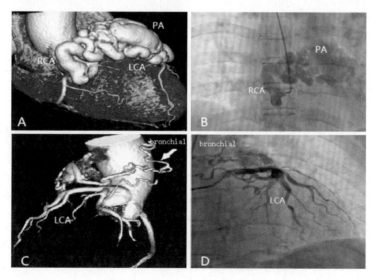

Figure 8-95 A & B: CT image showed tortuous and dilated vessels originating from both RCA and LAD. Angiogram showed the tortuous and dilated tract; C & D: CT image showed multiple tortuous tracts communicating with the bronchial artery (arrow). Angiogram showed these tortuous vessels from LCA, but the aneurysmal sac was not clearly visualized.

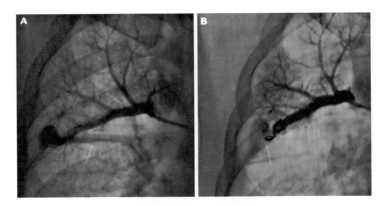

Figure 8-96   A: Before coil embolization of arteriovenous fistula in the right lung (red arrow). The venous phase of the fistula was also seen (yellow arrow); B: After coil embolization, the angiogram showed obliteration of the fistula (red arrow) with near obliteration of the fistula (yellow arrow).

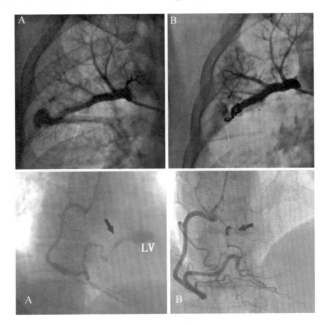

Figure 8-97   A: Selective ICA showed fistula (arrow) originating from the posterior LV branch with drainage into LV; B: Angiogram showed that fistula was embolized by 3 coils (arrow).

functional evaluation method for LCA-PA fistula. Ascending aortic angiography should be the first choice for cardiovascular examination, and selective ICA should be performed for large CAF (Figures 8-99, 8-100).

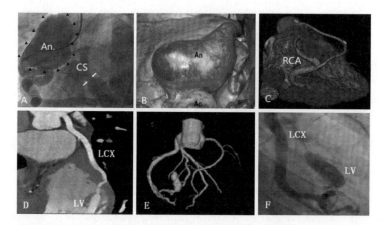

Figure 8-98 A: Angiogram showed the giant AN (black arrowheads) with fistula to CS (white arrows), originating from RCA; B: Intra-operative photograph of AN; C: Post-operative 3-D reconstruction image revealed no abnormal communication related to fistula and saphenous vein graft; D-F: LCX-LV fistula with the aneurysm.

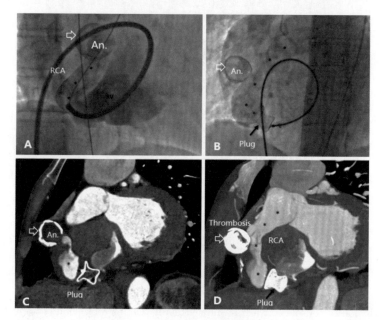

Figure 8-99 A: Angiogram revealed opacification of the artery (*) and the patent part of the saccular AN (white arrow) with opacification of RV; B: Amplatzer vascular plug (black arrow) was deployed at the distal drainage point. RCA angiogram revealed non-opacification of RV; C & D: Follow-up CTA image showed the vascular plug in-situ (black arrow) with complete thrombosis of the saccular AN (white arrow).

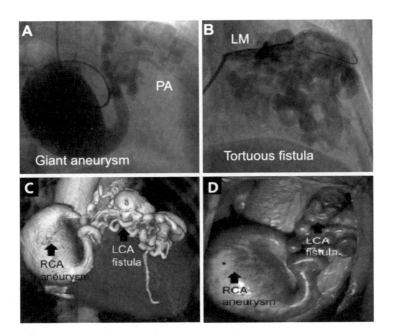

Figure 8-100　A: A giant AN originating from the proximal segment of RCA and draining into PA; B: LCA with drainage to PA near the ostial segment of LAD; C: Giant AN and fistula from the proximal RCA into PA and tortuous fistula from LAD into PA; D: Surgical image of the giant AN and torturous fistula.

Liu G and others retrospectively analyzed the clinical and imaging manifestations of 55 adult patients with congenital CAF among 32,114 patients with ICA. The results showed that the course of disease ranged from 2 days to 20 years, including 30 cases of precordial pain, 20 cases of chest tightness and shortness of breath on exertion, 1 case of back pain, 1 case of palpitation and 1 case of syncope; 11 cases could hear the murmur in the precordial area, and 44 cases had no prominent murmur; there were 29 cases of hypertension, 12 cases of diabetes and 18 cases of CAD; coronary angiogram showed that the fistula originated from LAD in 31 cases, LCX in 6 cases, RCA in 7 cases, LAD and RCA in 11 cases; there were 43 cases of fistula into PA and 18 cases of multiple fistulas. The authors believe that the clinical manifestations of congenital CAF in adults are complex, without apparent specificity, and are easily covered up by other heart diseases. ICA is the gold standard for diagnosing CAF and can provide detailed morphological and hemodynamic information of CAF (Figures 8-101, 8-102).

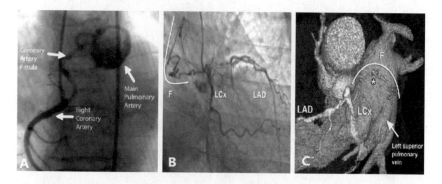

Figure 8-101   A: Angiogram of RCA-PA fistula; B: LCA-LA fistula; C: LCX-left superior pulmonary vein fistula.

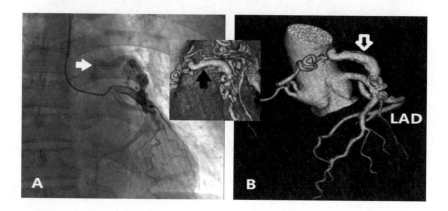

Figure 8-102   Angiogram and CTA of LAD-PA fistula.

Hayman S presented 2 cases where fractional flow reserve (FFR) was utilized to guide the management of CAF, an approach advocated in recent case studies. The authors suggest FFR may only be assessing the concomitant epicardial CAD rather than the degree of coronary steal and its routine use in this setting is not supported (Figure 8-103).

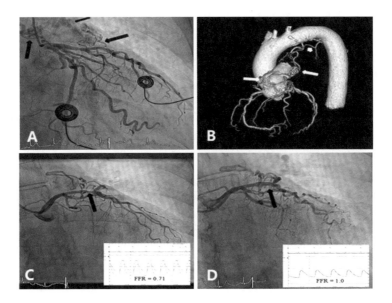

Figure 8-103   A & B: One case. A: Diagnostic angiogram showed CAF terminating in PA (small arrow) with origins arising from LM and LAD (large arrows); B: CTA confirmed these findings (large arrows) and revealed an additional fistula from the aortic arch (small arrow). C & D: Another case. C: Angiogram showed CAF and stenosis (arrow). D: Post-PCI with DES (arrow).

Huang Z presented the case of a female with typical palpitation and chest tightness due to the coronary steal phenomenon of bilateral CAPF. The fistulas were safely and successfully closed by coil embolization. The author also showed a new tool for the sophisticated evaluation of the hemodynamic significance of CAPF using FFR measurement. FFR, OCT, or IVUS, could be a promising means for the option of therapeutic regime of the CAPF (Figure 8-104).

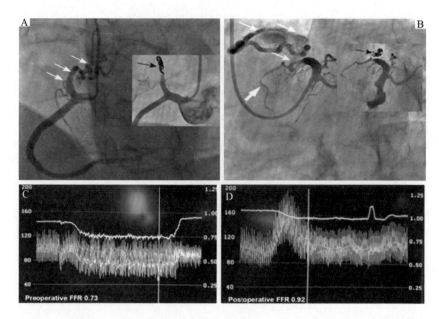

Figure 8-104 A: Angiogram demonstrated RCA-PA fistula (white arrows); B: Angiogram demonstrated LAD-PA fistula (small white arrows). Moreover, the angiogram demonstrated a poor development of the distal LAD (bold white arrows). Shunt between RCA/LAD and PA was blocked by coil embolization (black arrow); C & D: The FFR of pre- and post-operation in LAD.

Chapter IX   Diagnosis and differential diagnosis

Highlights

- CAF should be considered if there is palpitation, or exertional shortness of breath, 2-3/6 continuous murmur can be heard in the precordial area, and the location is lower than that of PDA. Retrograde ascending aortic angiography, CTA, and color Doppler Echo can confirm the diagnosis.

- The main diseases that need to be identified include PDA, AN rupture of the aortic sinus, aortic-pulmonary artery septal defect, VSD with aortic insufficiency, and LCA originating from PA.

- CAF is a rare congenital malformation that causes myocardial ischemia. However, a few cases also occur in the invasive examination, surgery, or trauma of the heart and coronary artery.

The clinical diagnosis needs to be combined with the patient's symptoms, such as palpitation, shortness of breath, chest tightness, and chest pain. On auscultation, two-phase murmur can be heard. At the same time, further combination with X-ray, ECG, treadmill test (TMT), Echo, CTA or MR, and ICA is the gold standard for diagnosis. ICA can distinguish the fistula, the degree of tortuosity, and whether there is coronary artery expansion, to make a diagnosis and guide the subsequent treatment, such as medicine, TCC, and surgery operation. The disease often causes the insufficient blood supply to the myocardium and angina pectoris. In severe cases, it can cause CHF (Table 9-1, Figure 9-1).

The diagnostic criteria of CAF usually include chest X-ray, ECG, CT/MR, PET or scintigraphy (SPECT), cardiac catheterization, or ICA (Figures 9-2, 9-3).

(1) Chest X-ray: Radiography can be used to diagnose CAF, which is a common imaging examination. Through this examination, the patient's

condition can be clearly defined and the extent of enlargement of RA or LA can be understood.

Table 9-1   Auxiliary inspection methods of CAF

Exam	Signs
Physical examination	Atypical systolic, diastolic or continuous murmur
ECG	Volume overload; Left or right ventricular hypertrophy
	Atrial fibrillation; Myocardial ischemia pattern
Chest X-ray	Cardiomegaly and pulmonary congestion
Echo	Enlargement of left or right chambers
	Defects in segmental or global ventricular function
	Origin or drainage sites of CAF using CDFI (rare)
TEE	Origin or drainage site of CAF using CDFI
	Localization of CAF; Useful intra-operatively to attest the closing
TMT	Ischemic pattern; Arrhythmia
CT	Anatomy of CAF (origin and drainage sites)
	Stenosis; Coronary steal phenomenon
MR	Anatomy of CAF; Ischemic myocardium (stress thallium studies)
SPECT	Myocardial ischemia
Catheterization	Anatomy (origin and drainage sites)
	Hemodynamic status of CAF; Stenosis; Treatment
IVUS/FFR/OCT	Hemodynamic quantification; Morphology of CAF

(2) ECG (Figure 9-4): Like chest X-ray film, CAF can not be determined by ECG. In other words, the diagnostic value of chest radiographs and ECG for CAF is limited. If LV and/or RV are overloaded during the examination, the CAF can be directly diagnosed.

(3) TTE can display CAF with hemodynamic significance, but it is unhelpful to determine the origin and termination site. TTE is sufficient to diagnose this disease in children. CDE is also helpful in identifying dilated or distorted arteries and in mapping blood flow. At the beginning and the end of the fistula, a larger flow than usual can be seen. In addition, inappropriate blood flow into RV or

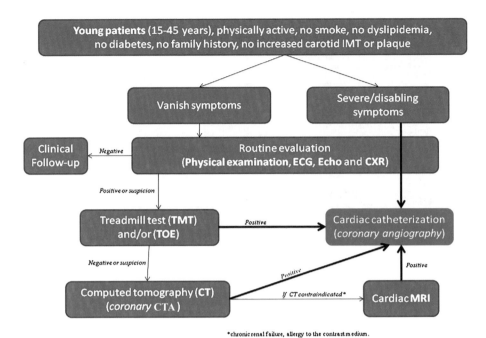

Figure 9-1   Suggested flowchart for faster CAF diagnosis.

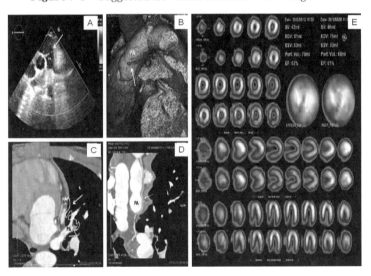

Figure 9-2   Multimodal imaging approach to study CAF. A: TTE showed an abnormal color Doppler flow draining into the main PA (arrow); B-D: CTA identified small and extremely tortuous fistula connecting the proximal part of LAD with PA; E: Stress myocardial perfusion scintigraphy was performed: after stress, no ischemic abnormalities were identified.

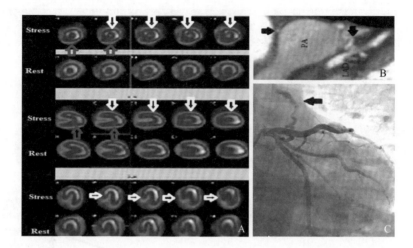

Figure 9-3   A: Stress myocardial perfusion imaging showed mild-moderate reversible cardiac perfusion defect in the territory of LAD (the anterior and anteroseptal walls, white arrows) and moderate reversible cardiac perfusion defect in the inferior wall (red arrows) and on rest SPECT images; B & C: CTA and angiogram showed the fistula (black arrow) between the proximal LAD and the main PA.

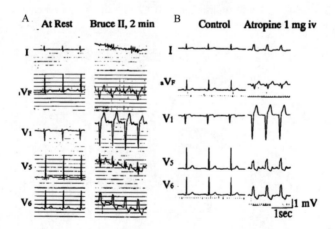

Figure 9-4   A 49-year-old male with chest pain both on effort and at rest. Tachycardia-dependent LBBB complicated with exertional angina. A: HR increment was induced by TMT using Bruce protocol; B: Intravenous (iv) Atropine. In either cases, LBBB appeared when the HR exceeded 85 bpm. Chest pain occurred simultaneously with LBBB.

LV can be seen by CDFI. TEE helps to assess turbulent blood flow in adults and delineates the origin and drainage site of the fistula (Figure 9-5).

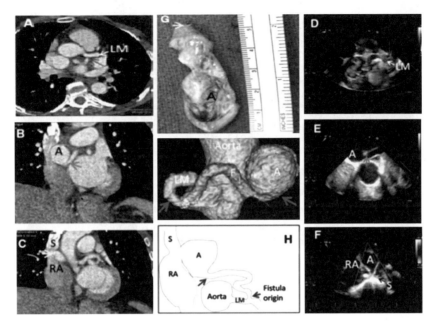

Figure 9-5　A-C: MDCT demonstrated CAF origin and connections; D-F: Multiplane TEE; G: Surgical specimen; H: Schematic diagram. The fistula origin (red arrows) was from LM. It connected (blue arrows) to an aneurysmal sac-like cavity, which ended (yellow arrows) by emptying into SVC.

(4) CTA/MR: Multi-slice spiral CTA and MR can clearly and accurately display the anatomic and pathological changes of CAF and its associated malformations, providing a sufficient basis for diagnosis. Cardiac MR can also be used to identify CAF (Figure 9-6). In recent years, coronary CTA is not only non-invasive but also has a higher detection rate than standard invasive ICA.

(5) Cardiac catheterization: Monitoring pressure and blood oxygen saturation in various parts of the heart can also identify CAF well. If the patient's CAF enters the right heart cavity, this examination will find that the blood oxygen content at the level of RA, RV or PA increases and determine the location of the left-right shunt. When the shunt is large, the patient's PA pressure may be slightly elevated.

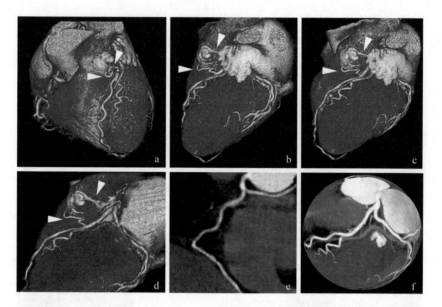

Figure 9-6　a-d: Contrast-enhanced retrospectively ECG-gated coronary CTA showed CAF arising from LAD with angiomatous plexus (arrowheads) draining into PA; e & f: CT images with curved multiplanar reconstruction (MPR) showed the 2 CAF.

(6) Angiogram: Patients with CAF can also be diagnosed by cardiovascular angiography. Suppose it is found that the contrast medium has dilated fiber bending, sometimes tumor-like dilated lesions, and the coronary artery enters the heart cavity. In that case, the situation can be clarified, and the specific location of CAF can be understood (Figure 9-7).

There is no doubt that coronary catheterization and subsequent ICA are the gold standards for diagnosing CAF. Overall, studies have shown that aortic root angiography should be performed first to help guide the next step of management. This initial step will help to select the most appropriate coronary artery for angiography. The next step is to perform selective ICA on each artery, with the aim of determining the starting and ending positions and estimating blood flow. In some cases, retrograde angiography can also be used.

De Doelder MS and others believed that multiple imaging examination methods plays an essential role in the diagnosis of CAF and reduction of

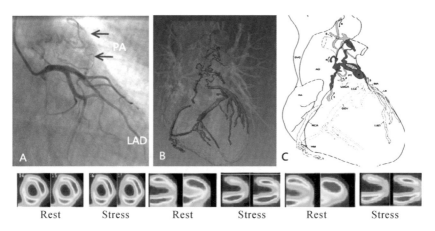

Rest   Stress   Rest   Stress   Rest   Stress

Figure 9-7   A: Angiogram of LAD and LM-PA fistula; B & C: Schematic representation of MDCT showed hexalateral CAF. These vessels bifurcated and anastomosed, and finally terminated into PA (asterisk); The next row: Myocardial perfusion imaging and PET/CT scanning demonstrated reversible myocardial ischemic changes in several segments.

misdiagnosis or missed diagnosis. Hong SM and others believed that no matter the current imaging progress, Echo had always been the most basic and accurate examination method for diagnosing CAF (Figure 9-8).

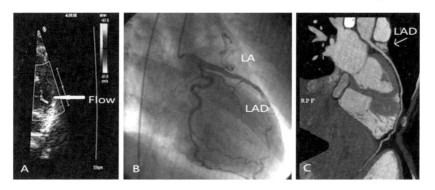

Figure 9-8   Imaging value of CAF. A: An abnormal blood flow was found through the pulmonary valve by Echo; B: Angiogram showed LAD-LA fistula; C: CT showed the tortuous LAD (arrow).

Based on the case history, signs, and auxiliary examination data, the diagnostic essentials of CAF include:

(1) Typical patients have clinical symptoms similar to angina pectoris. In

addition, some patients may have symptoms such as shortness of breath, fatigue, palpitation, and chest tightness on exertion. During the physical examination, asymptomatic patients may find continuous murmur in the precordial area with cardiac enlargement. If CAF is not operated or treated early, the symptoms and signs of cardiac insufficiency will gradually appear with age.

(2) The characteristics of chest X-ray film are cardiac enlargement, cardiothoracic ratio > 0.5, abnormal cardiac contour, abnormal vascular shadow visible in individual patients, and cardiac enlargement is out of proportion due to increased pulmonary blood flow.

(3) Older patients are often accompanied by LV hypertrophy, biventricular hypertrophy, or ST-T changes in ECG, and some patients may even have malignant events such as ventricular arrhythmia.

(4) Echo can find the opening of the dilated coronary artery draining into the abnormal cardiac cavity or blood vessel and measure the abnormal turbulence spectrum. In some patients, the location and size of the fistula can be determined by TEE. a. The origin of the involved coronary artery, fistula, and orifice was significantly dilated, and the inner diameter was more than 6 mm. b. Abnormal turbulence in the involved coronary artery, especially the high-speed turbulence signal at the fistula. c. Aortic and atrioventricular cavity dilatation and valvular insufficiency.

(5) On selective ICA, it can be seen that the thick and abnormal coronary artery is tortuous and coiled, and the branches that drain into the cardiac cavity or large vessels are diffusely or smoking-like developed.

(6) The main sign of CAF is cardiac murmur. If the loudest part of the murmur is located between 2-3 intercostals at the left edge of the sternum, it should be distinguished from PDA. In case of increased pulmonary blood and enlarged heart, it indicates that PDA is thick. The patient's murmur is loud, and the patient often has a history of pneumonia in childhood, but the patients with CAF have no obvious performance in this aspect; if systolic murmur and continuous murmur similar to VSD are heard at the left edge of

the sternum, it should be distinguished with PDA. The main points of differentiation are that the continuous murmur of patients with CAF has positional variation and lacks signs of pulmonary hypertension.

(7) Others: Some patients may have elevated myocardial enzymes, such as increased BNP levels in patients with CHF and increased CT_n-T, CK/CK-MB level in AMI.

The continuous murmur produced by CAF is similar to that of PDA, with main aorticopulmonary septal defects, ruptured AN of aortic sinus, high position of VSD with aortic insufficiency, pulmonary arteriovenous fistula, which is easy to be confused. The possibility of CAF should be considered in the differential diagnosis of cases with atypical symptoms. The following diseases should be distinguished from CAF:

(1) Kawasaki disease: Also known as cutaneous mucosal lymph node syndrome, its clinical manifestations are fever, lymphadenopathy, etc. Coronary arteries can dilate or form AN, but there is no arteriovenous and coronary-chamber communication (Figure 9-9A-D).

(2) Single AN: One or more segments of the coronary artery are swollen, usually located at the bifurcation of the coronary artery. RCA is common, and other coronary arteries can also occur. There is no communication between the involved coronary artery or cardiac chambers (Figure 9-9 E and F).

(3) The left and right coronary arteries originating from PA: CDE showed the continuous blood flow signal between the coronary artery and · PA, and coronary artery dilation and tortuosity (Figure 9-10).

(4) Aorta-LV tunnel: It is an extremely rare congenital heart malformation with an abnormal channel between aorta and LV. CDE showed a continuous blood flow signal from the aorta to the abnormal channel, and a diastolic blood flow signal was at the opening of LV.

(5) Aorticopulmonary septal defect: It is a rare congenital heart disease caused by abnormal development of the main aorta and pulmonary artery septum. The aorticopulmonary artery septum was interrupted continuously,

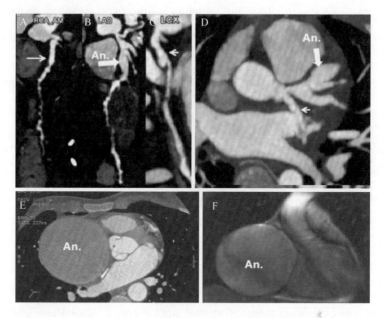

Figure 9-9 A-D: AN of RCA, LAD, D1, and LCX; E & F: CTA and MR of huge RCA aneurysm.

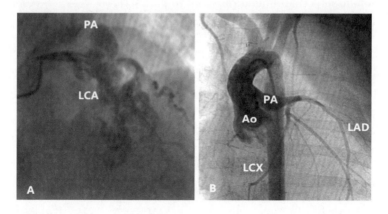

Figure 9-10 A: LCA-PA fistula; B: LCA originating from PA.

and CDE showed the continuous shunt signal from the aorta to PA.

(6) PDA: The murmur is high, located in the second intercostal space on the left edge of the sternum, and the shape of murmur is rhombus. Echo showed a channel between the main PA and the descending aorta with the left-right shunt. Ascending aortic angiography showed that PA and

descending aorta were developed simultaneously.

(7) Rupture of aortic sinus aneurysm: There is a history of sudden chest pain, and the course of the disease progresses rapidly. The murmur was located between the 3-4 ribs of the left sternal margin and was evident in diastole. Echo showed shunt between the highly dilated aortic sinus and the cardiac cavity. Ascending aortic angiography showed that the blood in the ascending aorta flows into the broken heart cavity.

(8) VSD combined with aortic insufficiency. The murmur is located in the 3-4 intercostals of the left sternal margin and is discontinuous. Right heart catheterization showed a shunt at the ventricular level. The ascending aortic angiography showed that the contrast medium flowed back from the ascending aorta into LV, and RV was developed simultaneously (Figure 9-11).

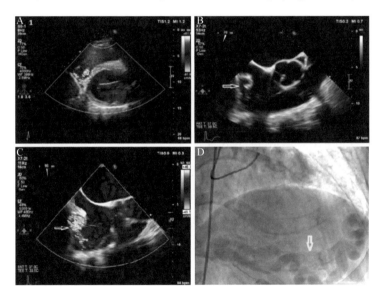

Figure 9-11   A-C: TTE and TEE showed LCX-RV fistula resembling VSD; D: ICA showed tortuous course of LCX (arrow).

According to the comprehensive symptoms, precordial murmur, X-ray cardiogram, ECG, and Echo, the diagnosis of this disease is not difficult, but it needs to be differentiated from other CHD. Atypical cases can be distinguished by ascending aortic angiography or selective ICA.

The evaluation of CAF begins with auscultation of persistent murmurs in the precordial region. The initial diagnostic examination may include chest radiography and ECG. Although these methods can not provide sufficient diagnostic evidence, they can help to find any subsequent complications. For example, ST segment changes on ECG may indicate AMI or chronic myocardial ischemia; Chest X-ray can assess the volume overload.

Studies have shown that TTE can show CAF with hemodynamic significance, but it is not helpful to determine the origin and drainage site. CDE can also identify dilated or distorted arteries and map the blood flow. At the beginning and end of the fistula, a larger flow can usually be seen. TEE helps assess turbulent blood flow in adults and delineates the origin and drainage site of the fistula.

There is no doubt that aortic angiography and subsequent ICA are the gold standards for diagnosing CAF. In general, studies have shown that aortic angiography should be performed first to guide the next step of management and select the most appropriate coronary artery for selective or superselective ICA. In recent years, it has shifted from ICA to CTA, and CTA scanning is the same as routine ICA.

Most cases of CAF were asymptomatic and diagnosed incidentally during a routine clinical examination. On physical examination, atypical systolic, diastolic, or continuous murmur can be heard occasionally. Typically, the continuous murmur is in the shape of crescendo-decrescendo but louder during diastole. On the contrary, most of the other continuous murmurs reach their peak intensity at the time of the second sound. There is a correlation between the drainage site of CAF and the site of the loudest intensity of the murmur. When CAF drains into RA, the murmur is the loudest along the sternal border. If CAF drains into PA, the murmur is the loudest at the second intercostal space to the left sternum, and if CAF drains into LV, the murmur is the loudest near the apex. PDA, ruptured sinus of Valsalva, internal mammary-PA fistula, intracardiac mass or tumor (Figure

9-12), and aorta-LV tunnel might be considered as differential diagnosis. Color-flow mapping may be useful to confirm the diagnosis, which should be confirmed by ICA.

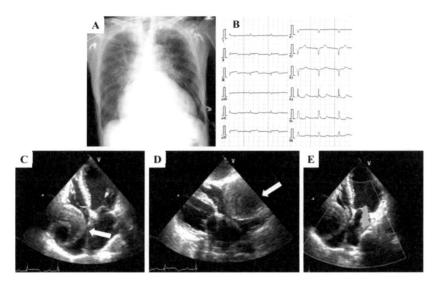

Figure 9-12   Chest X-ray film (A), ECG (B) and Echo (C-E) of the patient with AN. ECG showed ST elevation in lead Ⅱ, Ⅲ, and aVF; Echo showed an enlarged mass lesion measuring nearly 80mm (white arrow).

Echo can provide some helpful information if CAF is suspected, such as coronary artery dilatation, termination chamber, turbulent flow, volume overload, and kinesis of LV segments. Thanks to its non-invasive, Echo is also useful after CAF treatment to monitor the status of CAF and LV wall. Moreover, the severity of blood shunt could be determined by CDFI. In addition, Echo could confirm the existence of CAF during prenatal diagnosis, and pulsed Doppler could reveal the blood flow signals through the fistula.

TEE gives a better view of the morphology of the fistula concerning its origin, course, and termination. It can be helpful to determine the precise drainage site when surgical closure is required. TEE is an invaluable tool, as precise termination points are often not detectable through pre-operative ICA.

Echo diagnosis of CAF should be distinguished from aortic regurgitation

(AR) and VSD:

(1) Echo shows the turbulence signal on the aortic valve in diastole in AR patient, while the high-speed turbulence signal in the whole period and the origin from the coronary artery in CAF patient.

(2) Echo shows continuous interruption of the ventricular septum in VSD patients, and CDE shows right-left shunt or bidirectional shunt during systole.

The followings should be noted about Echo diagnoses CAF:

(1) Although most of the involved coronary arteries are dilated and tortuous, a few are normal, and the fistulas are short and easy to ignore by Echo. For example, on the Echo examination, the abnormal blood flow signal can be found in the cardiac cavity or large blood vessels through multifacet and multi-angle exploration supplemented by CDE. The possibility of CAF should be considered if the patient has no septal blood flow, large artery shunt, and CS aneurysm rupture or valve regurgitation.

(2) Most orifices of CAF drain into the right heart system, but the incidence of drainage sites into PA varies greatly. The results of surgery and ICA show that the incidence of CAPF is high, while the Echo literature reports that CAPE is less.

(3) When CAF enters LV, the systolic pressure of LV is the same as that of aorta, and the shunt may not be observed. The shunt is only seen in the diastole, shown as the diastolic turbulence spectrum.

(4) CAF are mostly single, and there may be multiple fistulas. On Echo examination, the doctors should carefully observe the abnormal blood flow signals, origins, drainage sites of CAF, and anatomical relationship between normal and abnormal arteries.

The reasons why Echo's diagnosis of coronary-PA fistula is easy to be missed:

(1) It may be related to a small fistula and less shunt.

(2) It is easily confused with the main aorticopulmonary septal defect, PDA, and other diseases.

(3) Improper instrument conditions, inappropriate color pulse repetition

frequency (PRF), and insensitivity to low-speed blood flow.

(4) The patient's sound transmission condition is poor.

Second-level examinations include MDCT or MR (Figure 9-13). CT is superior to Echo in overweight patients with an excellent anatomical delineation. The presence or absence of coronary stenosis can be determined with CT as well as coronary steal phenomenon detection. Cardiac MR of CAF with relevant shunting is feasible and could provide additional data with a better anatomical view. Its greatest limitation, however, is the determination of distal coronary course. Therefore, the latest technique could be more helpful in evaluating the distal CAF, collateral vessels, and coronary origin outside the normal sinuses (e. g. from PA).

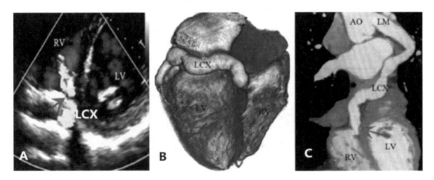

Figure 9-13   Echo and CT images of LCX-RV fistula.

Furthermore, visualization of the posterior descending branch takes work. Exercise tests and myocardial perfusion scans are valuable methods for assessing myocardial ischemia related to CAF. The radionuclide examinations can generally dictate whether invasive treatment is required or not. If the patient remains asymptomatic with limited ischemic territory (<10% of LV), medicine is the first-line treatment.

ICA remains the primary diagnostic technique for CAF detection and hemodynamic evaluation; moreover, it can achieve interventional closure with proper devices. In addition, an intravascular ultrasound (IVUS), FFR and OCT analysis may provide more information about the pathophysiology of the fistula.

Surguladze G and others believe that the CAF should be vigilant if a large mass in the heart is found. In 1995, Said SAM. reported that 26% of intracardiac masses were later confirmed as CAF during ICA (Figure 9-14).

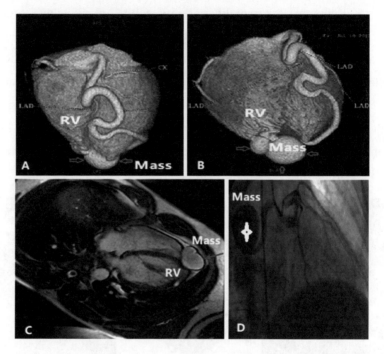

Figure 9-14   A-C: CT and MR images of LAD-RV fistula with an apical visible 4.5 cm × 3.2 cm × 3.0 cm mass; D: Angiogram showed coronary artery pseudotumor formation.

By 2022, Sokmen A Fournier JA and others reported less than 20 cases of coronary-coronary fistula, which should be distinguished from CAD with collateral formation (Figures 9-15, 9-16).

Xu Z, Shi D, and others analyzed the clinical data of congenital CAF in middle-aged and older people, and summarized the characteristics of these special patients:

a. There were chest distress attacks similar to angina pectoris;

b. Physical examination showed no positive signs. Unlike CAF in children and young people, no obvious cardiac murmur was found;

c. Coronary artery dilatation and multicolored blood flow mosaicism were found in a few cases;

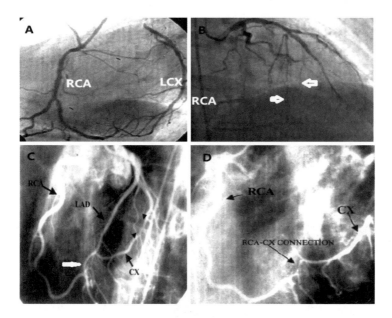

Figure 9-15   A: RCA-LCX fistula; B: RCA occlusion with collateral circulation formation from LAD; C & D: RCA-LCX connection.

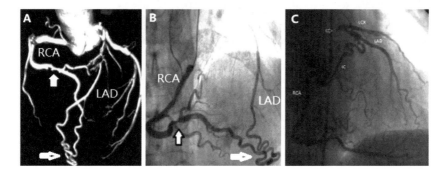

Figure 9-16   A & B: CT image and angiogram of RCA-LAD fistula; C: Angiogram of RCA-LM fistula.

    d. No positive findings were found in ECG, treadmill test, and Holter;

    e. There were no significant cardiovascular risk factors.

The authors believe that the late onset of symptoms in middle-aged and elderly patients with CAF might be related to the small fistula and shunt flow. The clinical symptoms are similar to angina pectoris, which may be related to the increase of vascular resistance and the lower resistance of

CAF, so the coronary steal phenomenon was aggravated. Middle-aged and elderly patients with CAF and chest tightness or chest pain are easily misdiagnosed as CAD.

Clinicians should not forget the diagnosis of CAF while considering the diagnosis of CAD, and selective ICA should be actively considered. With age, patients with CAF can be complicated with serious incidents such as myocardial ischemia, IE, AN, and even rupture. Therefore, once diagnosed, it should be treated actively, including surgical ligation and TCC, and the prognosis was good (Figure 9-17).

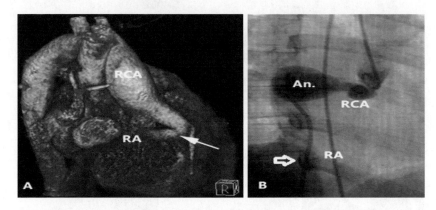

Figure 9-17 CT image and angiogram of RCA-RA fistula with AN.

Ge L and other scholars believe that diagnosing CAP is not difficult, and the key is to identify the related symptoms of pericardial tamponade as soon as possible (Figure 9-18). When the patient is suspected of pericardial tamponade, the doctors should exclude reasons that may cause low blood pressure, such as bleeding at the puncture site, retroperitoneal hematoma, myocardial ischemia or AMI, contrast agent allergy, and vagal reflex. In addition to Bp monitoring, cardiac shadow and patient condition observation, Echo is significant in the diagnosis and treatment of CAP. In the pericardial tamponade caused by CAP, the delayed attack is easily ignored. The incidence of delayed pericardial tamponade is about 5%– 10% , and the cause is mainly related to guidewire (61.5%). Chua YL analyzed the clinical data of 13,888 patients with PCI from 1992 to 2006, including 21 patients with CAP

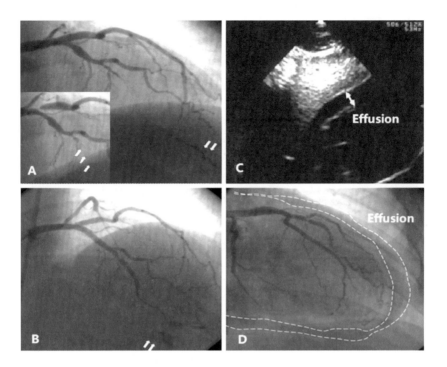

Figure 9-18   A: Total occlusion of the middle and distal LAD (arrow), and the guidewire and microcatheter were used to try to open the occlusive lesion; B: The distal LAD was perforated and the contrast agent penetrated into the pericardial cavity (arrow); C: Immediately, bedside Echo revealed a large amount of pericardial effusion (1.9 cm) and RV diastolic collapse; D: The patient has sinus tachycardia and blood pressure drop (60/40 mmHg), indicating pericardial tamponade. During ICA, a large amount of pericardial effusion was found in the pericardial cavity (within the white dotted line). The operation was terminated. The patient was given 50mg Protamine intravenously, 500 ml blood was drawn out by emergency pericardial puncture, and Dopamine 7 μg/kg/min was given simultaneously. Despite continuous pericardial drainage and administration of positive inotropic drugs, the patient's condition was still worsened, and the blood pressure still fluctuated at 80/40 mmHg. Considering the possibility of RV perforation, the treatment strategy was changed, pericardial drainage was stopped, rapid volume expansion was performed, and plasma was infused. The patient's blood pressure gradually recovered to 120/70 mmHg. Echo showed that RV collapse was significantly improved, and the pericardial effusion volume was significantly reduced. The patient was sent to CCU for follow-up 24 hours later. Echo showed that RV was not collapsed, a small amount of pericardial effusion, and hemodynamics were stable. The patient was discharged 2 days later.

and 2 patients (10%) with delayed pericardial tamponade. The foreign studies showed that the occurrence time of delayed pericardial tamponade was mostly 4.9 ± 3.4 (2 – 15 hours) hours after the operation. Therefore, in clinical practice, if a patient has CAP, regardless of the type, it is necessary to follow-up with Echo regularly after the operation. CAP may lead to death (< 9%), AMI (4% – 26%), emergent operation (24% – 36%), and blood transfusion (34%). If the patient uses a GP Ⅱb/ Ⅲa inhibitor, the risk of death will increase by 2 or more times.

According to observation and research of Ellis GS. , the severity of adverse events in hospital are closely related to the classification of CAP: death and AMI are mainly limited to the patients with type Ⅲ CAP, and the majority of patients with pericardial tamponade and emergent CABG are also type Ⅲ CAP (63%). The incidence of emergent CABG and pericardial tamponade in patients with type Ⅰ and type Ⅱ CAP is significantly reduced. The observation and study of Dipper EJ. also confirmed Ellis's findings: the prognosis of type Ⅱ perforation is relatively good, there is no death and emergent CABG, and only 5. 3% of patients need pericardial puncture. Type Ⅱ perforation occurred in 73.7% of the patients using GP Ⅱb/ Ⅲa inhibitor, 21.1% received Protamine treatment, 15.8% received platelet infusion, and 26.3% had low pressure expansion of the balloon. Even so, the prognosis of type Ⅱ perforation was still good.

On the contrary, the prognosis of type Ⅲ perforation is more dangerous. Although very active treatment measures (64.3% Protamine, 50.0% platelet transfusion, and 85.7% low pressure expansion of balloon), the mortality of type Ⅲ perforation is still as high as 21.4% , the incidence of pericardial tamponade is 42.9% , and the emergency CABG is 50.0% . Stankovic G. also pointed out that the death of patients during hospitalization and emergency CABG were related to type Ⅲ coronary perforation.

Chapter X   Treatment

Highlights

- CAF patients with CHF, angina, or recurrent IE should undergo surgical treatment. If the shunt flow is small and asymptomatic, it can be observed temporarily, and the operation can be performed when there is a surgical chance incidentally.

- Patients without other cardiac malformations requiring surgical correction and iatrogenic CAF caused by traumatic or coronary intervention should be performed TCC.

- Cases with difficulty in TCC can choose surgical treatment, including direct suture, direct coronary artery repair, and intracardiac fistula repair.

- Most asymptomatic CAF does not need treatment, just follow-up observation and necessary examination. Excessive medical treatment harms such patients, but doctors have an impulse to treat any abnormality of the heart actively.

1. Treatment principle

The standardized treatment of CAF has not been established. Patients with clinical symptoms, such as increased ventricular filling load, CHF, insufficient myocardial blood supply, and IE, should consider surgical treatment once the diagnosis is clear. There are different opinions on the surgical indications of infants or children with small CAF and shunt volume, Qp/Qs less than 1.3, and clinically asymptomatic. Some scholars believe that long-term follow-up observation can be carried out for these patients. When CAF has expanding trend or clinical symptoms, surgical treatment can be considered. Another opinion is that the possibility of spontaneous closure of CAF is scarce, the surgical treatment is simple and safe with good long-term effects. In order to prevent various complications that may occur after growing up, surgical treatment should be performed in childhood after the diagnosis is determined (Figures 10-1, 10-2).

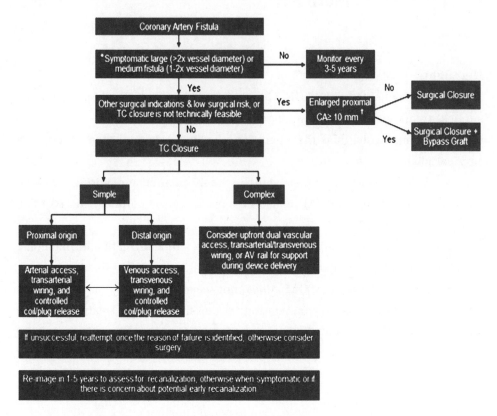

Figure 10-1 Detailed algorithm of CAF evaluation and management.

Currently, the conventional treatment methods for CAF include conservative treatment, TCC, and surgical operation (Table 10-1). Based on the fact that CAF is mostly asymptomatic, the first-line treatment is essentially medical therapy with follow-up for life.

For CAF patients with chest pain or CHF, the principle should be to relieve symptoms and wait for surgery. Patients with CHF usually choose diuretics, vasodilators, β-blocker, ACEI/ARB and digitalis. Sometimes, Phentolamine can be used to reduce pulmonary hypertension, and β-blocker has obvious effects on relieving angina pectoris. In the case of AMI, intravenous thrombolysis or emergent PCI and double antiplatelet drugs can be used. Antibiotics can be used to prevent IE in some cases. Due to the low incidence of coronary-LV fistula, there is still a lack of standard treatment.

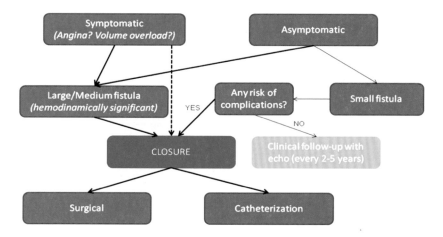

Figure 10-2   Simplified algorithm for management of CAF. The dotted arrow indicated the possibility of treating.

Table 10-1   Indications of the various modalities of treatment for CAF

Conservative	Small CAF
	Medium-sized asymptomatic CAF
Surgery	Cases requiring concomitant CABG, valve repair or replacement and anomalies needing repair
	Distal CAF
	High-velocity CAF
	CAF with tortuous courses or complex communications
	Those with multiple drainage sites or a "fistula lake"
	Signs of volume overload
	Proximal CAF with large AN
TCC	Proximal CAF with single-site drainage
	Distal narrowing of CAF with device access feasibility
	Non-tortuous vessels and the absence of vessels that could be embolized accidentally
	Serious cardiac comorbidities

Cheng TO believes that β-blocker and calcium channel antagonists could be treated conservatively for these patients with coronary artery-fistula. Ge L and other scholars believe that some CAP could be treated with drugs such as Protamine.

Concerning children, especially those over 5 years old, elective closure for some clinically apparent fistulas should be performed, even if the patient remains asymptomatic. Late stenosis secondary to intimal hyperplasia represents a significant complication reported in children, which could increase the risk of AMI. Spontaneous thrombosis of CAF with secondary closure has been reported on rare occasions, mostly for small fistula in infants younger than 2 years. Patients with small, asymptomatic fistula should not be treated but managed by clinical follow-up, including Echo every 3-5 years (Class Ⅲ, Level of evidence C). In this case, the patient should undergo treatment only if the patient is at high risk of IE or if follow-up over time is not feasible, as well as if the case undergoes an invasive cardiac procedure for other reasons.

Currently, 50%–60% of AN are reversible at 1-2 years after the onset, most likely if they are small, RCA involved, the age of onset is less than 1 year, and they are fusiform and located distally. Patients with large fistula have a higher risk of increased progression to stenosis with a worse prognosis for giant AN (>8 mm). Medical therapy is recommended and should be administered for at least 6-8 weeks or until the documented regression of AN. In the case of giant AN, antiplatelet agents with or without Warfarin and low molecular weight Heparin should be administered. β-blocker is useful for the reduction of myocardial oxygen consumption.

The same drugs are also employed in adults, based on the size of the fistula, the number of involved arteries, and the presence of multiple giant AN with or without angiographically documented coronary obstructions. Finally, in all patients with CAF, regardless of the size and type of fistula, prophylaxis for IE is recommended, although this decision should be individualized.

Small fistulas may be hemodynamically insignificant and may even close spontaneously. Percutaneous TCC with coil embolization is preferred, but surgical ligation is also an alternative. ACC/AHA guideline for the diagnosis and treatment of CHD in adults (Class Ⅰ, Level of evidence C) recommends that the patients with small and medium-sized CAF with myocardial ischemia, arrhythmia, unexplained ventricular systolic or diastolic dysfunction, or cardiac enlargement, or endocarditis and asymptomatic large CAF, should be treated with catheterization or surgery.

Yan R described a 55-year-old man who was asymptomatic and diagnosed with RCA-RA fistula and giant AN. Because the AN was in the distal right posterior descending coronary artery, RCA ligation and fistula occlusion through RA were performed without CPB. The AN was excluded without impacting the myocardial blood supply, and the patient was exempted from a lifelong anticoagulation regimen. The follow-up revealed favorable outcomes, and the patient's life expectancy was improved (Figures 10-3, 10-4, and 10-5).

The conservative treatment of medicine is mainly the prevention and treatment of IE and CHF; alternative interventional treatment methods include controllable/uncontrollable coil embolization, covered stent implantation, self-expanding umbrella occluder, etc. For extremely low mortality, patients with clear evidence of shunt should be treated with surgery, while those without clinical symptoms or evidence of shunt should be treated conservatively. The operation methods can be selected according to the pathological conditions: (a) Coronary artery ligation; (b) Suture closure of CAF; (c) Coronary artery incision and closure; (d) Closure of fistula through cardiac incision. The first 2 surgical methods do not need CPB, while the latter 2 must be operated under CPB. The surgical treatment of CAF is effective, but patients with giant AN have a higher risk of operation, and the mortality is about 2%. The complication rate of post-operative AMI was 3%–6%, and CAF recurred in 4% of patients. After long-term follow-up, the clinical symptoms disappeared, and the cardiac function

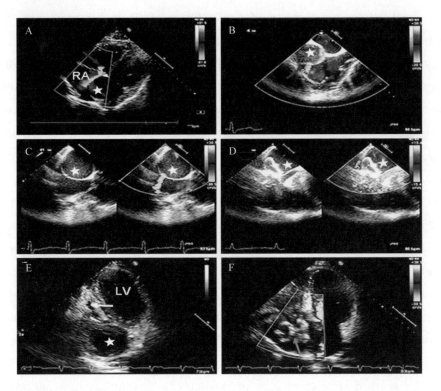

Figure 10-3   Echo findings before, during and 3 months after operation.
A & B: Pre-operation Echo demonstrated giant RCA aneurysm (white star) with
fistula to RA (blue arrow); C & D: Intra-operative TEE showed 30 mm ASD
occluder (red star) was placed; E & F: Three months post-operation, TTE revealed
mural thrombosis in AN, and no residual shunt between RCA and RA was found.
The visual segment of RCA was still dilated (white star).

returned to normal.

Armsby LR and others believe that TCC is safe and effective, can
significantly shorten the hospitalization time, and has fewer post-operative
complications, which is worthy of recommendation. Surgy should still be
recommended to patients who have failed medical treatment or TCC, and
need surgical treatment for cardiovascular diseases. In order to prevent the
thrombosis of coil or occluder after TCC, Aspirin, Clopidogrel, or
Rivaroxaban should be taken orally for more than 3-6 months after the
operation, and follow-up should be strengthened.

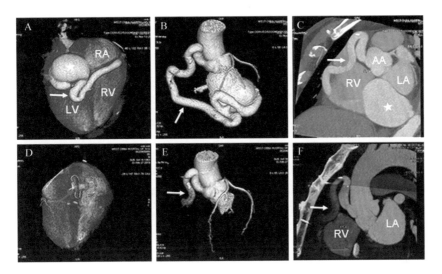

Figure 10-4　Pre- and post-operative CT findings. A-C: Pre-operation CT showed tortuous and dilated RCA (white arrow) and the diameter increased to 11 mm, giant AN (white star) originating from the distal RCA and draining into RA; D-F: Three months post-operation, there was no displacement of the occluder (red arrow) and the thrombus formed at the distal end of RCA was undeveloped.

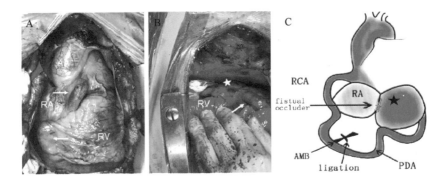

Figure 10-5　A: Intraoperation confirmed tortuous and dilated RCA (white arrow); B: Aneurysmal dilation behind RV (white star); C: A schematic diagram of the operation: RCA was significantly tortuous and dilated, the ligation was performed 3 cm at the distal end of the acute marginal branch (AMB), and then the fistula was occluded through RA.

Post-CAF treatment sequela include thrombosis and MI, revascularization, persistent coronary dilatation and remodeling. The large and distal CAF may be at the highest risk for coronary thrombosis post-closure. The optimal treatment approach to various morphologies of CAF at various ages remains to be determined.

Treatment and further management are only applicable to the following patients:

a. Hemodynamically significant left-right shunt;

b. CHF with LV volume overload or LV insufficiency;

c. Myocardial ischemia.

2. TCC

Although the surgical repair was once considered the treatment method for CAF, TCC has recently become the preferred treatment. In catheter plugging, the purpose is to embolize the artery at the farthest end of CAF and the closest to the termination site. The basic principle is to ensure that the myocardium supplied by the coronary artery is still perfused. In addition, the shunt of blood through the fistula is reduced. Some mechanisms of embolization are achieved by using a detachable balloon or steel/platinum micro-coil. After TCC, the next step is to perform post-operative ICA to ensure the success of embolization, and a small residual fistula or branches may be seen.

In the past, surgical repair was used to treat CAF, in which the internal closure was the goal. However, surgery is considered to be associated with a higher degree of fistula recurrence. Therefore, catheter plugging is preferred (Figures 10-6, 10-7, Table 10-2, 10-3, and 10-4).

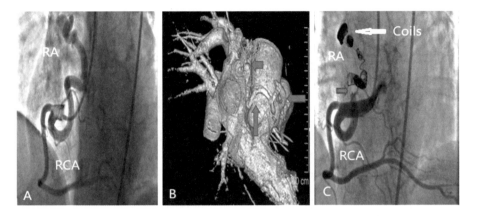

Figure 10-6   Comparison of RCA-RA fistula pre- and post-TCC. A & B: Pre-operative angiogram and CT image; C: Angiogram of post-TCC.

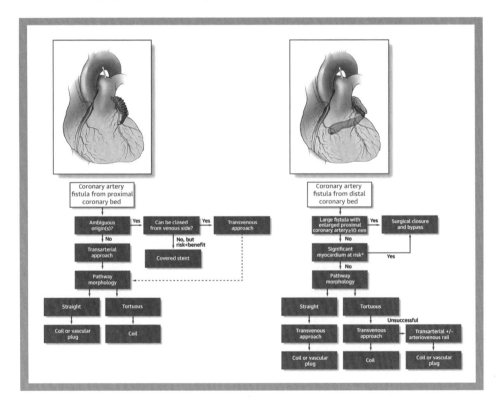

Figure 10-7   Algorithm of CAF closure for fistula originating from proximal and distal coronary bed. * Significant myocardium at risk was defined by the number and size of branches that might be compromised with CAF.

Table 10-2 Indications and contraindications for CAF closure

Indications for TCC or surgery

Symptomatic medium or large CAF ∗

—Evidence of ischemia in the feeder artery territory

—Arrhythmia thought to be related to CAF

—Endarteritis

—Vessel rupture

—Cardiac chamber enlargement

—Ventricular dysfunction

∗ A medium fistula is defined as a vessel that is ≥ 1 to 2 times the largest diameter of the coronary artery not feeding CAF. A large fistula is defined as a vessel that is more than 2 times the largest diameter of the coronary artery not feeding CAF.

Indications for TCC

—Congenital CAF with obvious symptoms, without other CHD requiring surgical correction

—Iatrogenic CAF caused by trauma or PCI; fistulas with less vascular expansion and distortion, easy to reach safely and can be clearly developed

—For non-multiple CAF, TCC for single CAF is effective; stenosis of CAF and tumor-like expansion of fistula

—There is no thrombosis in the fistula, and CAF has only one outlet and is smaller than the inlet

—In a few cases, one or more branches (mostly septal branches) of the coronary artery form multiple microvascular networks connected to the cardiac cavity, and can be blocked with covered stent

---

Relative indications for TCC

Small CAF have little blood flow and no obvious clinical symptoms, and some scholars believe that interventional treatment is not necessary

---

Contraindications for TCC and indications for surgery

—At the distal of the coronary artery to be blocked, there are important coronary artery branches (side branches), where the myocardial blood supply is normal, and the blocking is easy to cause AMI and death

—The involved coronary artery is extremely tortuous or too huge to achieve satisfactory occlusion effect

—The right cardiac angiography suggested right-left shunt and severe pulmonary hypertension

—Severe infection within 1 month before occlusion

—For those with several fistulas that are not suitable for interventional therapy or multi-vessel blood supply; patients with tortuous coronary artery; coronary bifurcation greater than 90 degrees makes it difficult to locate the catheter

---

Table 10-3   Equipment list used for device delivery

· 100 cm guiding catheter

· Microcatheter

· Guide extension catheter

· 125-cm, 5-F multipurpose diagnostic catheter (for telescoping technique)

· Hydrophilic-coated sheath, such as Flexor shuttle sheath (Cook Medical) or Destination sheath (Terumo Medical)

· Deflectable sheath, such as small- and medium-curl Agilis sheath (Abbott Vascular) or Dexterity sheath (Spirus Medical)

· 0.014-inch coronary wire

· 0.035-inch hydrophilic guidewire (regular and exchange length)

· 6-F Goose Neck (Medtronic) or En-Snare retrieval catheter (Merit Medical)

Table 10-4   Compatibility, advantages, and disadvantages of commonly used CAF closure devices

Type of Device	Examples	Compatibility	Advantages	Disadvantages
Vascular plug	AVP-II and AVP-IV	Guide or shuttle sheath	Good for large CAF Repositionable Accelerated thrombogenicity	Large delivery catheter profile need for additional support to deliver
Pushable coil	Nester coil (Cook Medical) Tornado coil (Cook Medical)	0.018- to 0.035-inch microcatheter, depending on required coil size 0.018- to 0.035-inch microcatheter depending on required coil size	Good for large CAF Repositionable Accelerated thrombogenicity Easier to deliver	Large delivery catheter profile Need for additional support to deliver
Detachable coil	Retracta (Cook Medical) Ruby (Penumbra) Azur (Terumo Medical) Concerto(Medtronic)	0.035-inch internal diameter, 2.5- to 2.9-F, 100- to 150-cm microcatheter such as the Cantata microcatheter (Cook Medical) 0.025-inch internal diameter Lantem microcatheter (Penumbra) 0.018- to 0.035-inch internal diameter Progret microcatheter(Terumo Medical) 0.017- to 0.021-inch internal diameter	Good for small, tortuous vessels Accelerated thrombogenicity	Embolization risk with pushable coil, lower risk with detachable coil given controlled release Inability to reposition with pushable coil Multiple coil needed to provide full seal of the flow
Stent graft	JOSTENT GraftMaster (Abbott Vascular) PK Papyrus stent (Biotronik)	6-F guide for 2.8 ~ 4.0mm 7-F guide for 4.5 ~ 4.8mm 5-F guide for 2.5 ~ 4.0mm 6-F guide for 4.5 ~ 5.0mm	Treat plexiform fistula	High thrombosis risk

In the first 6 months after cardiac catheterization, patients should take antiplatelet and anticoagulants in all cases. Clinicians should attach great importance to this point, CAF closure procedures can be complicated by post-procedural AMI.

In some cases, an experienced interventional cardiologist embolizes the CAF using coil or other device without the need of surgery. Use of TCC device is reserved for CAF with favorable characteristics, such as non-tortuous coronary artery, fistula with distal narrowing, and no additional cardiac defects necessitating surgical intervention. However, because the TCC approach can produce some complications, and there are also some requirements for CAF, many patients have to undergo surgical closure as the preferred therapy.

The results of all techniques for CAF closure are acceptable with total mortality of < 1% and low complications. The choice of the technique for CAF closure depends on its morphology, course, tortuosity, and the presence of aneurysmal dilatation of the vessel. In fact, in the case of a single fistula, an elective coil seems to be preferable over surgical ligation.

In the 1990s, new approaches were attempted with the use of coils or stents that cause thrombosis of CAF via the percutaneous approach. TCC is associated with lower incidence of complications compared to surgery: fewer bleeding, lower infection, rare arrhythmia and myocardial ischemia (Figures 10-8, 10-9).

The main advantage of TCC over surgery is the avoidance of CPB or median sternotomy and the related iatrogenic complications, and others include the reduction of the costs, quick recovery, and good cosmetic results, which is the important factor especially in young patients.

The techniques for TCC of CAF include various types of coils (Gianturco and polyester covered stainless steel coils), umbrella-shaped devices, detachable balloon, vascular plug, covered stent, glue, and histoacryl resin or other occlusive oil, which are mainly used in smaller CAF. The Amplatzer duct occluder is an adaptive device for bigger CAF, which required the

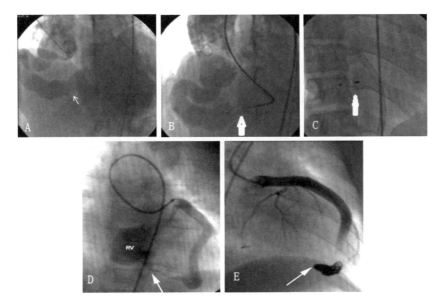

Figure 10-8   A-C: TCC of large congenital CAF using wire-maintaining technique (12 mm VSD occluder); D & E: TCC of LCA-RV fistula (coils).

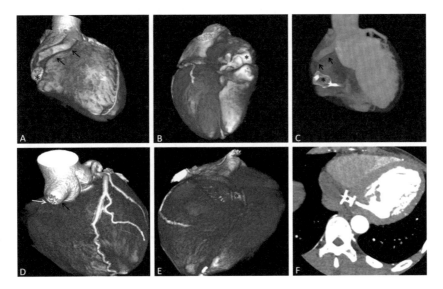

Figure 10-9   3-D CT scan of 2 patients at 12-month follow-up. A-C: No thrombus in the proximal cul-de-sac off RCA (black arrow); D-F: Thrombus (yellow arrow) had formed in the proximal cul-de-sac off RCA (black arrow).

drainage to be large enough to allow the passage of the long sheath. Encouraging results come from the use of Cook coil by arterial approach and Nitinol duct occluder by venous approach.

TCC of CAF is feasible in most patients. However, extreme vessel tortuosity may cause this approach to be unsuitable, as well as multiple drainage sites. On the other hand, TCC is preferred in cases of proximal CAF with single drainage site, non-tortuous vessel, distal narrowing of CAF with an accessible way for closure device, absence of important branches that could accidentally be embolized, and absence of other cardiac disorders or high peri-operative surgical risk (Figure 10-10).

With increased experience, newer devices and techniques, TCC of CAF is being confirmed as a successful therapeutic strategy. To avoid short/long-term complications, it would be preferable to perform regular angiographic follow-up to check the results of TCC.

Transcatheter embolization could bring about some complications during operation including spasm of coronary arteries or CAP and arrhythmia. Malpositioning or proximal extension of coil or device may obstruct side branches and myocardial ischemia. Incomplete occlusion by coil and the presence of a foreign body can increase the risk of IE.

Xiao Y documented TCC approaches for CAF and devices election based on fistula origin. The choices of TCC technique and device are primarily determined by the heterogeneous anatomic characteristics of CAF (Figures 10-11, 10-12, 10-13, and 10-14).

Neylon A described the case of an elderly female with large symptomatic CAF that was treated using the percutaneous approach with a vascular plug (Figure 10-15).

Xian X summarized the experience in treating 40 patients of CAF by using Guglielmi detachable coils. No procedure-related complications occurred. Intra-operative angiography showed that residual shunt completely disappeared in 12 patients (30%), and blood flow was significantly decreased in 28 patients (70%). All patients were followed-up, and neither

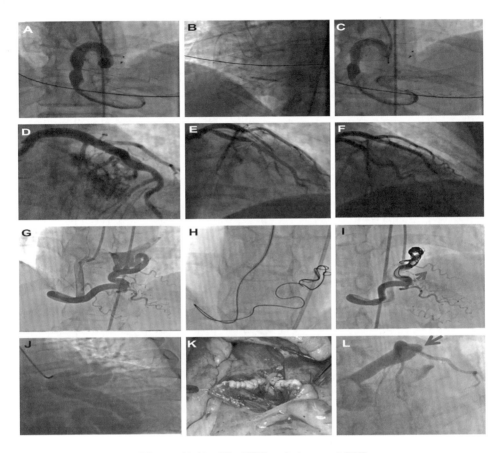

Figure 10-10   The TCC techniques of CAF

A: A patient presenting with inferior STEMI after successful closure of the distal coronary fistula. ICA revealed disruption of flow to the distal RCA with large thrombus; B: The patient was treated with balloon angioplasty and thrombectomy; C: Subsequent ICA revealed minimal improvement of flow to the distal vessel. The patient was treated with anticoagulant; D-F: A case of a 48-year-old woman with complex plexiform LAD-LV fistula. The flow into the fistula was terminated with the deployment of two 5.0 mm × 16 mm covered stents. The double-layered stents increased the risk for stent thrombosis; E: The patient presented a few days later with anterior STEMI due to stent thrombosis (red arrow); F: The patient was successfully treated with balloon angioplasty and DES placement; G-I: A 45-year-old woman with RCA enlargement and a large fistula originating from the distal RCA into CS. Angiogram showed complete release of the detachable coil, abolishing flow to CS; J-L: A 56-year-old woman with CHF and a large LCX-CS fistula. The patient underwent surgical fistula closure without CPB and developed ventricular fibrillation due to inferior STEMI. Angiogram revealed thrombotic occlusion of the ectatic LCX (red arrow).

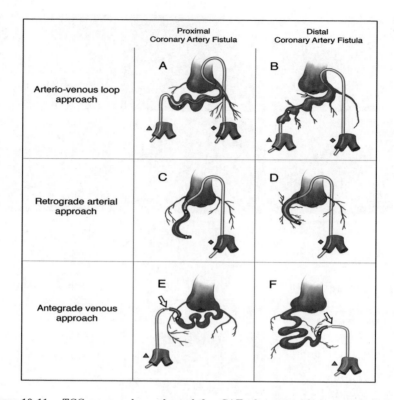

Figure 10-11 TCC approaches adopted for CAF closure with a potential site of occlusion based on the type of CAF. Yellow asterisk indicated potential sites for device delivery and occlusion of CAF. The use of co-axial catheter system was represented by the arrows. The use of venous system for device delivery was represented by the blue color triangle. Red color diamond signified use of the arterial system.

complications such as recurrent shunt and ischemia nor stenosis and occlusion of related arteries, or fistula cavity rupture occurred. The use of Guglielmi detachable coil in the interventional treatment of CAF is safe and effective, although its long-term effect needs to be further verified.

Yakut K aimed to review the treatment options and long-term problems of patients diagnosed with CAF. From 2000 to 2018, the medical records of 56 CAF patients (33 males and 23 females) were retrospectively reviewed. TCC was performed in 10 patients, while CAF was corrected surgically in 5 patients. Vascular plug was deployed in 6 patients, platinum coil was used in

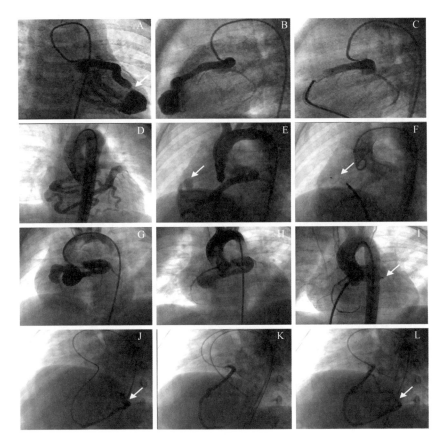

Figure 10-12   TCC of CAF using arterio-venous (AV) and arterio-arterial (AA) loop approach. A-C: AV loop approach for large LAD-RV fistula. There was narrow constriction proximal to aneurysmal dilatation (A, arrow) and device closure was proximal to the aneurysmal neck (C) using a delivery system from the venous end; D-F: AV loop approach for large LAD-RV fistula (E, arrow) and final delivery of duct occluder (F, arrow) at the drainage site; G-I: AV loop approach for large LCA-RA fistula with successful closure using duct occluder at its proximal end (I); J-L: AA loop approach for medium-sized LCA-LV fistula. After creating an AA loop (K), duct occluder II was delivered at the drainage point (L, arrow).

3 patients, and platinum coil with tissue adhesive was placed in 1 patient. Early complications were seen in 2 patients during TCC and 1 patient during surgery. There were no instances of death or late complications in patients treated surgically or with TCC.

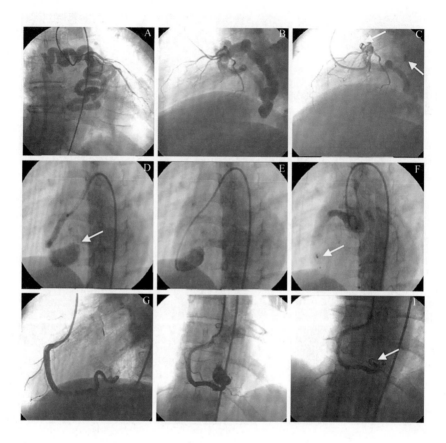

Figure 10-13 TCC of CAF using the retrograde arterial approach. A-C: Medium-sized LCA-SVC fistula. Two coils (C, arrow) were delivered with the retrograde arterial approach using co-axial guide/Glide catheter system. There was quite sluggish flow in this long cul-de-sac with dye note ven-reaching the coils—a potential for large thrombus; D-F: Large RCA-RV fistula with aneurysmal end (D, arrow), device deployment at the neck of AN (F, arrow) was performed; G-I: Medium-sized RCA-CS fistula. Two coils were delivered at the drainage point (I, arrow).

CAF is usually asymptomatic, and medical processing with long-term follow-up is the first-line treatment. And for those CAF that cause hemodynamically significant shunt, chamber enlargement, or visible symptoms should be closed at an early age. TCC is a safe treatment option for CAF that may be performed with a high success rate and stabilization

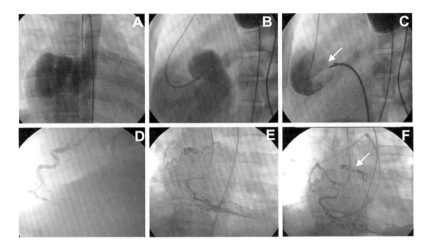

Figure 10-14   TCC of CAF using the antegrade venous approach. A-C: Large tortuous RCA-RA fistula. XDO device was delivered at the drainage site (C, arrow); D-F: Small RCA-PA fistula. Two coils were delivered at the distal part of the fistula (F, arrow).

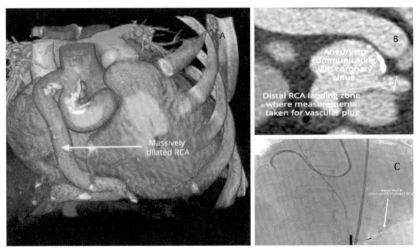

Figure 10-15   A: 3-D CT reconstruction demonstrated giant RCA; B: CT image demonstrated distal AN communicating with CS and landing zone for vascular plug (arrow); C: AVP Ⅱ in distal RCA prior to deployment (arrow).

(Figures 10-16, 10-17). Also, it should be known that surgery may be performed effectively with lower complications. Because complications can develop in treated and untreated patients of all ages, follow-up should be accepted during the patient's lifetime.

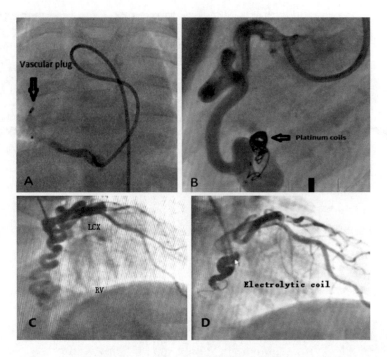

Figure 10-16 A: Vascular plug placed in the distal LCX of a one-year-old child was seen, and no residual shunt; B: In a 14.5-year-old patient, 5 platinum coils placed in RCA was seen, and no residual shunt; C: Angiogram showed LCX-RV fistula; D: Electrolytic coil placed in LCX.

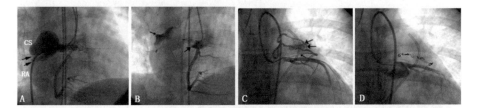

Figure 10-17 A: ICA showed RCA fistula with AN, and 2 exit sites (arrows) near the junction of SVC and RA; B: Amplatzer vascular plug (large arrows) was placed proximally in the fistula and another Amplatzer vascular plug (small arrows) was placed in the largest exit in hopes of reducing the propagation of thrombus that could form in the AN sack; C: ICA demonstrated small, tortuous fistula from the proximal LAD to PA. There were multiple openings into PA (arrowheads); D: Multiple microcoils had been deployed to occlude the fistula.

3. Surgery

Once diagnosed, some patients with CAF should be given appropriate treatment including surgery. With age, patients with obvious shunt have more complications, such as CHF, IE, AMI, or fistula rupture, and sudden death of unknown cause during strenuous exercise, so they should be treated surgically in childhood. Furthermore, this disease combined with other CHD can be treated by surgery at the same time.

(1) The definite surgical indications are those patients with CHD or angina pectoris. However, there is still controversy about the surgical treatment of asymptomatic patients. Early treatment, especially for asymptomatic adolescent patients with large CAF and AN, closing the fistula can eliminate the shunt, improve myocardial blood supply, and prevent possible symptoms and complications in the future. In other words, patients with CAF and AN, or related symptoms and high-level shunt, should be treated as soon as possible. The severe compression of AN on the myocardium and distal coronary artery results in myocardial ischemia, expanding heart, and even CHF. Thrombosis and thrombus shedding in AN can lead to coronary embolism and AMI.

(2) The purpose of surgical treatment of congenital CAF is to selectively close the fistula without damaging the normal coronary circulation. Some CAF can be closed without CPB, and others usually need to be repaired under CPB, especially in the following cases:

a. Fistula behind the heart, which is difficult to expose, such as RVOT, CS, or ventricular posterior wall;

b. When the coronary artery is significantly dilated or combined with AN, the exact location of CAF can not be determined from the heart surface, so it is necessary to open the dilated coronary artery or AN;

c. Close the fistula from the cardiac cavity;

Common operations and their choices are as follows:

—Ligation or sutured (Figure 10-18): However, due to the concern of AMI, some doctors gave up this operation. Surgical ligation at the drainage site of CAF should be the preferable way of treatment, avoiding the occurrence of myocardial ischemia.

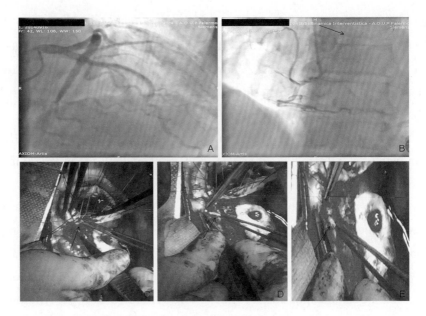

Figure 10-18　Fistula closure by surgical ligation of the drainage site was successfully performed with symptoms relaxation. A: ICA showed ectatic LCA; B: CAF (arrow) that arose from the RCA draining in PA; C-E: During surgery for the replacement of aortic valve, the operative fields confirmed the presence of small CAF (arrows) arising from RCA and draining to PA that was isolated and ligated closer to the drainage site.

　　—Inferior tangential suture of a coronary artery: For the lateral fistula originating from LM, several tangential mattress sutures and padded mattress suture ligation through the myocardium can prevent tearing of the myocardium and firmly close the fistula.

　　—Intracardiac fistula repair: CAF behind the heart is not easy to be exposed, and it is necessary to open and close the fistula through the cardiac cavity under CPB.

　　—Open and repair of dilated coronary artery or AN: If patients with significantly dilated arteries or complicated with huge AN, which can not determine the fistula from the appearance of the heart. And the surgeon can open AN vertically with CPB, and repair it under direct vision.

　　—Some CAF can be treated by closing their distal ends through the opened PA or aorta. The last technique is simultaneous valve surgery with additional CABG.

Residual shunt and myocardial ischemia are the most common complications, and the early incidence is about 4% and 3.7%, respectively. After mattress suture or patch repair, the incidence has decreased in recent years. If the above complications occur, they can be diagnosed by intra-operative Echo and ECG, and then accept the appropriate medical or surgical treatment.

If the lesion is not suitable for transcatheter intervention, surgery is required, including suture ligation without CPB, and aneurysmectomy with closure of the fistula. Early and late mortality are low, and risk factors for death and ventricular dysfunction are related to coronary artery insufficiency and AMI after fistula ligation or aneurysmectomy.

Yim D and others effectively summarized their experience spanning over 3 decades in the management of CAF. They described 3 techniques of surgical treatment (Figure 10-19).

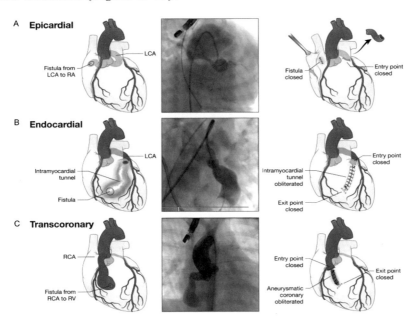

Figure 10-19   The epicardial, endocardial, and transcoronary methods of the closure of CAF.

—Epicardial: Dissection and mobilization of CAF with suture epicardial closure of the proximal and distal points of the fistula. Temporary occlusion with a tourniquet under continuous ECG monitoring preceded permanent closure of CAF to detect myocardial ischemia before closure.

—Endocardial: Closure was performed where the fistula was opened, and the lumen was sutured from the inside.

—Transcoronary: The aneurysmatic proximal RCA was opened, and the fistula was closed through the coronary artery.

The choice of endocardial, epicardial, or transcoronary closure is guided by the fistula anatomy and course. There is no preference for one technique over another. If cardioplegia is administered, a good myocardial delivery can be achieved by a simple trans-epicardial finger compression of CAF. However, cardioplegic arrest is not always required.

With various advancements in surgical techniques and tools, minimally invasive approaches have been used to treat CAF, especially in children. In some centers, it is the preferred strategy for treating CAF, except in cases of multiple CAF or patients requiring concomitant repair of other cardiac anomalies. In these centers, minimally invasive surgery (MIS) is reportedly associated with lower post-operative pain scores, faster recovery, and shorter hospitalization.

In 2014, Mitropoulos in Korea may be the first group to describe the left anterior mini-thoracotomy for ligation of CAF. MIS can be performed using one of several described approaches based on the location of CAF.

—Subxiphoid mini-thoracotomy with a 3 cm skin incision and resection of the xiphoid.

—Parasternal mini-thoracotomy through a 3–3.5 cm skin incision placed on the right or left, based on the fistula location.

—Partial inferior sternotomy using a 3.5 cm incision followed by division of the sternum up to the insertion of the fourth or fifth rib, depending on the CAF location. Care is taken to avoid injury to the internal mammary artery.

For patients with AN formation, Inoue H and others suggest that patients with small shunt, small AN size, or high surgical risk could be treated with interventional therapy, and the rest should be treated with surgery (Figure 10-20).

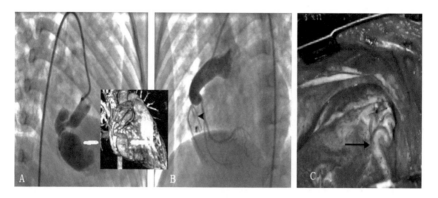

Figure 10-20   Pre- and post-TCC (A & B) and surgery field of RCA-RV fistula with AN (C).

Bloomingdale R reported a 34-year-old pregnant woman who presented with recurrent pericardial effusion and then was diagnosed with RCA-CS fistula. Her CS was significantly dilated due to the stenosis of CS ostium (Figures 10-21, 10-22).

Huynh KT reported the demographic, clinical, echocardiographic, and angiographic characteristics of CAF in patients encountered over 24-year and compared the short-term outcomes between surgical and TCC. The majority of fistula in this study originated from RCA and terminated in RA or RV.

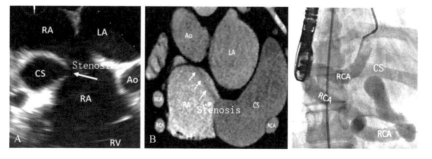

Figure 10-21   TEE (A), CT and Cardiac catheterization (C) of RCA-CS fistula showed the accelerated flow (B, negative washout, arrows) through CS ostial stenosis (dotted arrow).

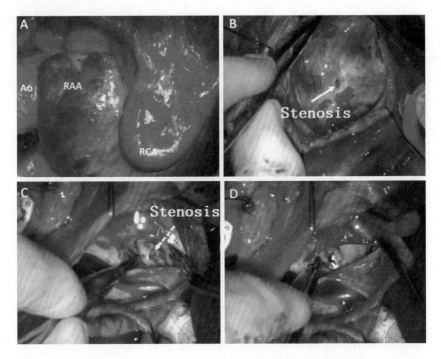

Figure 10-22   Intra-operative fields. A: RCA was severely dilated; B: Right atriotomy showed severe stenosis (arrow) of CS ostium; C: After resection of CS ostial stenosis, RCA-CS fistula opening (dotted arrow) was identified inside CS; D: The fistula was closed with mattress suture.

Transcatheter and surgical closure are both relatively safe and effective, with the potential for shortening the length of hospital stay following TCC. Uchino M reported 2 rare cases of aneurysmal CAF originating from LCX but treated with different surgical approaches. Surgical repair aims to prevent coexisting AN from rupturing, relieve adverse effects by AN compression, and prevent high-output CHF by significant shunting. To achieve these objectives, fistula closure with AN resection is required. Understanding the entire coronary artery is essential for determining surgical strategy. In the case of AN located proximal to LCX or extending to LCX, simple AN closure can cause AMI in the posterior LV wall. In the cases of CAF with large AN, it is difficult to detect the distribution of the coronary artery branches by ICA because of the contrast medium washout into the fistula and stagnation effect in AN. MDCT is more valuable than ICA in identifying the overall coronary vessel and drainage site of the fistula. The surgical strategy should be individualized and selected based on carefully evaluating of the pathological conditions and CAF anatomy. In particular, the intra-operative occlusion test is a useful diagnostic modality in determining the need for additional coronary revascularization (Figure 10-23).

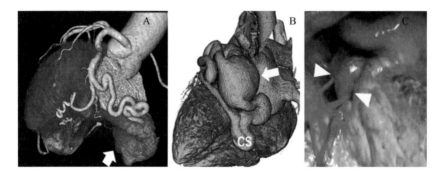

Figure 10-23   A & B: MDCT images showed abnormal AN from LCX to LA; C: Intra-operative fields.

4. Treatment of CAP and others

CAP is an infrequent complication, but it is still associated with high morbidity and mortality in patients undergoing PCI. It is critical for interventional cardiologists to take precautions to avoid this complication. It is more important to recognize it early if it occurs and to be familiar with the universal and specific management algorithms.

(1) Immediate low-pressure balloon expansion: The first step after diagnosis of CAP is to stop extravasation with inflation of the balloon (balloon:vessel size = 1:1) proximal to the site of perforation for about 5-10 min at low pressure (<8 atm). The maximum tolerated time to occlude coronary artery without causing significant myocardial damage is about 20 min. Therefore, repeated 5-10 min inflations can be done until either successful sealing of the perforation or evidence of significant ischemia.

(2) Specific management for distal-vessel CAP: In the case of distal vessel CAP, deployment of the covered stent in the main vessel at the ostium

of the perforated branch to occlude the origin or material (coil, autologous fat, gelatin sponge, etc.) embolization of distal vessel can be attempted.

(3) The embolization techniques: Guide catheters, thrombus aspiration catheters, over the wire (OTW) balloons, or microcatheters.

(4) Specific management for septal or epicardial collateral perforation: Uncommon during CTO intervention and are usually managed conservatively.

(5) Anticoagulant reversal: This is a crucial and the most important aspect of managing CAP. However, if done prematurely, it may precipitate life-threatening thrombotic complications and/or make it difficult to drain the pericardial fluid.

Ge L. proposed the treatment principles of CAP:

(1) Closed perforation.

—The balloon is extended and stuck under low pressure for a long time;

—Implantation of JoMed covered stent;

—Spring coil implantation;

—Gelatin sponge packing;

—Anhydrous alcohol ablation (PTSMA);

—Others (surgery, follow-up, etc).

(2) Maintain hemodynamic stability.

(3) Pericardial puncture drainage and autotransfusion.

(4) Hemostasis: Protamine neutralizes Heparin; fresh plasma or whole blood transfusion.

After the above medical treatment, 60%–70% of the patients do not need surgery. One thing we must remember is to avoid pressing the heart and perform emergent surgery if necessary.

The origin of the bronchial artery varies greatly. The ectopic bronchial artery originating from the coronary artery may participate in hemoptysis as an abnormal responsible vessel, which may cause the coronary steal phenomenon. The treatment process of coronary-bronchial artery fistula is shown in Figure 10-24.

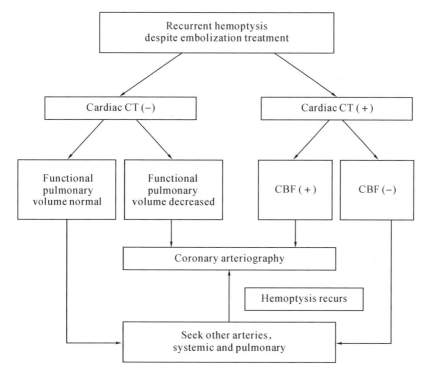

Figure 10-24   Diagnosis and treatment process of coronary-bronchial artery fistula (CBF) with hemoptysis.

Section I   TCC

In 1983, Reidy JF first reported TCC for CAF. After occlusion, the left-right shunt was reduced so that myocardial perfusion was restored to normal. It was a non-surgical method for occluding CAF and was considered an effective and minimally invasive treatment. The success rate reported in the literature was very high (Figures 10-25, 10-26). The comparative study of TCC and surgical results showed no significant difference in the early efficacy, complication, and mortality. The safety and effectiveness of the 2 methods supported the selective treatment of clinically significant CAF in children.

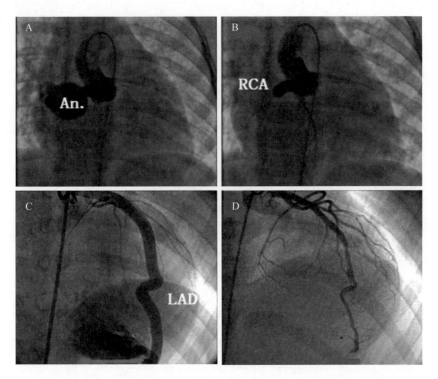

Figure 10-25   A & B: Large proximal RCA-RA fistula. Occlusion was obtained with 12 mm Amplatzer vascular plug; C & D: Large LAD-LV fistula. Occlusion was obtained with releasable balloon, and remodeling was observed 1 year after occlusion (D).

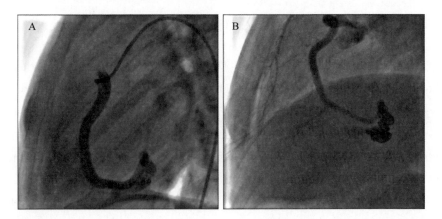

Figure 10-26   Large distal RCA-RV fistula. Occlusion was obtained with coils, and remodeling was observed 17 months after occlusion (11 coils) with minimal recanalization (B).

Pre-operative preparation:

(1) Signed the informed consent: Explain the patient's condition, necessity of the operation, and various possible complications during the operation, and complete the signing procedure.

(2) Pre-operative drug application: Including intravenous antibiotics, hydration, sedative half an hour before operation and selection of appropriate anesthesia. Patients with cardiac insufficiency should performed TCC after cardiac function improved.

(3) The femoral artery and vein were punctured, the sheaths were placed respectively, and heparinization was performed. If necessary, the bilateral femoral arteries should be ready for puncture. One side is used to deliver the occluder, and another is used to observe the final outcomes and coronary blood supply by angiography after occlusion.

(4) Cardiac catheterization: Left and right cardiac output, left-right shunt flow and pulmonary vascular resistance were calculated.

(5) Ascending aortic angiography: Observe the origin and direction of CAF and the site of the remote entrance, and perform selective left or right coronary angiography for determining the relationship with normal coronary artery (Figure 10-27).

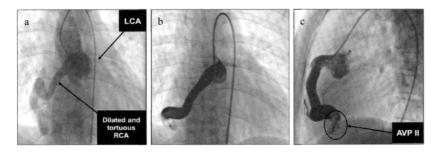

Figure 10-27   a: Ascending aortogram demonstrated dilated and tortuous RCA-RV fistula; b & c: Selective RCA angiograms demonstrated complete occlusion of CAF with AVP Ⅱ.

Çalik AN performed percutaneous closure of complex fistula that originates from all coronary arteries and drains to PA (Figures 10-28, 10-29).

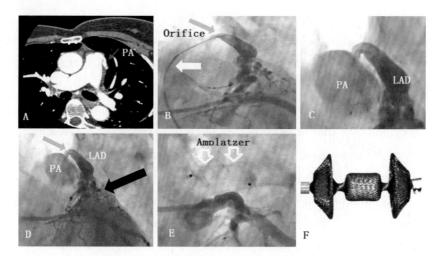

Figure 10-28 A-D: MDCT and ICA of the fistula; E: The anatomical conformity of the fistula and device; F: Amplatzer duct occluder Ⅱ device.

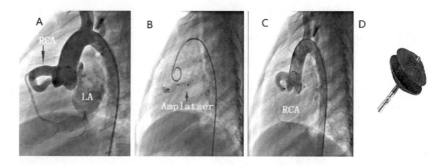

Figure 10-29 A: Ascending aortic angiogram showed dilated RCA-LA fistula; B: The fistula had been closed with Amplatzer duct occluder (arrow); C: Angiogram demonstrated that there were no obvious residual shunt after releasing the occluder; D: Amplatzer duct occluder Ⅱ device.

Zhang G and others reported the application of the interlock detachable coils system for occlusion of CAPF (Figure 10-30).

Lee W reported a 5-year-10-month-old boy who was diagnosed with CAF at birth. The follow-up TTE showed persistent CAF and progressed dilatation of LCA (Figure 10-31).

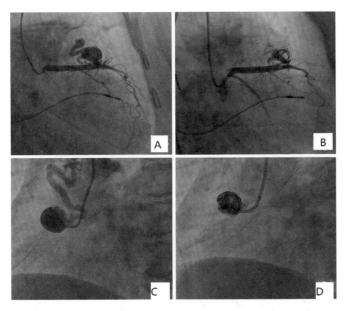

Figure 10-30   A & B: pre- and post-occlusion with interlock detachable coils(IDC) for LAD-PA fistula; C & D: Another patient of RCA-PA fistula.

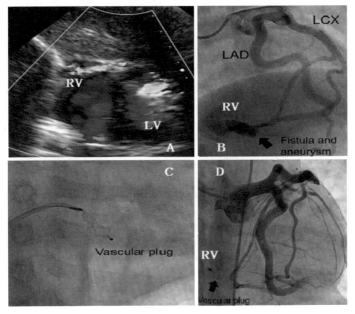

Figure 10-31   A: The flow of CAF to RV; B: CAF draining from the distal LCX to RV with AN formation (black arrow); C & D: Amplatzer vascular plug was used to close CAF via the antegrade method.

The key to the success of TCC technology is to find the fistula, and select the appropriate delivery route and embolic material according to the anatomical type of CAF (size, shape, origin, drainage site and single or multiple fistulas), the course of coronary artery and whether there are related collateral vessels, to block the fistula and prevent myocardial ischemia. Kim H reported a case of LAD-PA fistula closed with coils (Figure 10-32). Kassaian SE reported the experience of treating CAF with a covered stent (Figure 10-33).

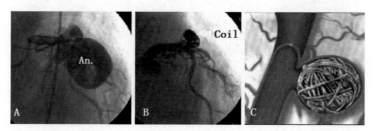

Figure 10-32 A & B: Pre- and post-TCC of LAD-PA fistula; C: Sketch map of TCC with coils.

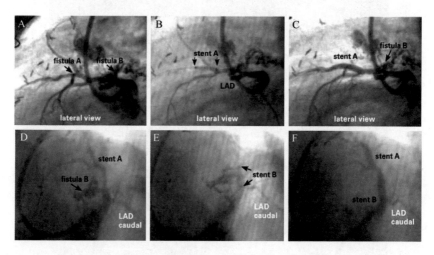

Figure 10-33 Treatment of LAD-PA fistula with a covered stent. A: 2 fistulas before stent implantation; B-E: Implantation process of 2 stents; F: Final angiogram.

For patients with stenosis of CAF, small and narrow coronary arteries, the common methods are steel wire and platinum mini-coil plugging; for patients with coarser coronary fistula, an occluder is selected. Davis JT pointed out that the residual blind end or bag after TCC would be the source of potential emboli and the cause of sudden death. Therefore, it was suggested that patients should take Aspirin and other antiplatelet agents regularly after the operation to prevent fatal embolism. Pedra C reported 2 cases of CAF blocked by interventional method (Figures 10-34, 10-35).

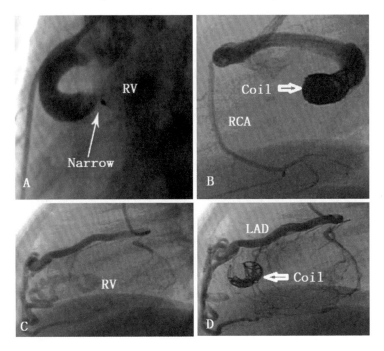

Figure 10-34   A & B: TCC of RCA-RV fistula with coils; C & D: TCC of LAD-RV fistula with coils.

At present, the most common approaches to TCC include antegrade occlusion via an artery and retrograde occlusion via a vein (Figure 10-36).

TCC occlusion test:

(1) Occlusion test is an essential step in the process of TCC.

(2) Use a balloon to completely block the CAF in advance, and observe the patient for more than 15 minutes. If ECG shows obvious depression or elevation of ST segment and inversion of T wave, or severe ventricular arrhythmia, or the patient has myocardial ischemic manifestations and cardiac dysfunction, the test should be stopped immediately.

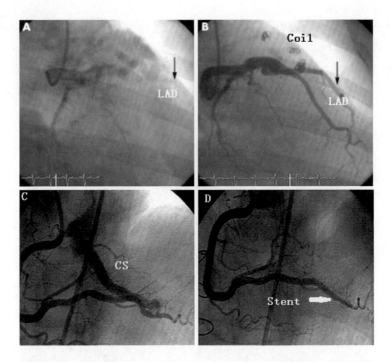

Figure 10-35 A & B: TCC of LAD-PA fistula with coils; C & D: TCC of RCA-CS fistula with a covered stent.

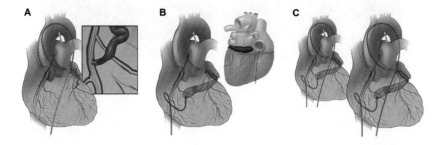

Figure 10-36 TCC Techniques. A: Transarterial approach. The coronary vessel was intubated, and the fistula was wired from its origin. The delivery catheter could then be delivered to the fistula over a wire for device deployment. The occlusion device was then deployed and released; B: Transvenous approach. The fistula termination site was intubated with the delivery catheter. This catheter was advanced over a wire to the appropriate landing zone. The occlusion device was then deployed and released; C: Arteriovenous (AV) loop approach. In large and tortuous fistulas, AV rail could be formed with the aid of a snare device to maximize support for catheter and device delivery.

(3) If the above symptoms such as myocardial ischemia occur, retract the spring coil or occluder, and readjust the occlusion position or device. If the patient still has the above conditions, the surgery should be terminated.

Device selection (Figures 10-37, 10-38):

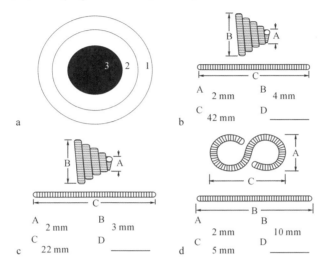

Figure 10-37   Sketch map of coils. a: Cross section of the coaxial delivery system; b & c: Cone-shaped Vortx-18; d: S-shaped Complex Helical Fibered Platinum Coil-18 followed by the Coil Pusher-16 in the central core.

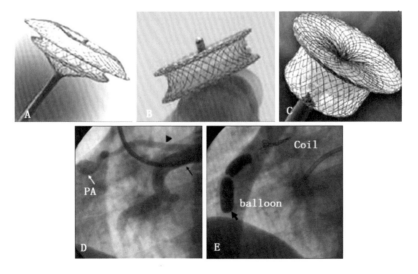

Figure 10-38   Amplatzer duct occluders and detachable balloon.

There are many kinds of embolic materials, such as detachable balloon, stainless steel spring coil, controllable coil, electrolytic detachable coil, PDA occluder (Amplatzer vascular plug, AVP, 4-16 mm in diameter), and covered stent with various chemical materials. At present, a controllable coil is used in interventional therapy, and the narrowest part of CAF is the best position for closure. If the angiogram shows no narrowest part of CAF, the occluder should be placed at the distal site, so as not to affect the normal coronary artery branches. If the narrowest part is ≤ 3 mm, the spring coil can be used for closure. The size of the spring coil according to the shape of CAF should be greater than 10%–20% of the diameter; it is recommended to use the Amplatzer duct occluder if the narrowest part is > 3 mm. Depending on the shape of the fistula, PDA or VSD occluder (generally greater than 2-4 mm in diameter) can be selected.

The spring coil is mainly used for small CAF. Its advantages show that the diameter of the delivery catheter is small, it can be directly delivered through the femoral artery with minor damage to the blood vessels, and the operation is relatively simple. Its disadvantages show that the closure of the large CAF is incomplete or unreliable. Covered stents are often used to occlude the multiple small vessel networks connecting with the coronary artery and the cardiac cavity; the Amplatzer PDA, VSD mushroom and umbrella-shaped occluder or plug are mainly used for relatively large coronary fistulas. Their advantage is good controllability, but they usually need to be inserted through the femoral vein.

Mullasari AS reported a case of CAPF with CHF treated by a covered stent (Figure 10-39A, B). Godart F reported a case of applying a detachable balloon to block LAD-RV fistula (Figure 10-39C, D).

In the past 40 years since 1983, the interventional treatment of CAF has been chiefly reported as coil closure, such as controllable and uncontrollable Gianturco coil. Jaiswal A reported 1 case of LAD-PA fistula blocked with coils (Figure 10-40).

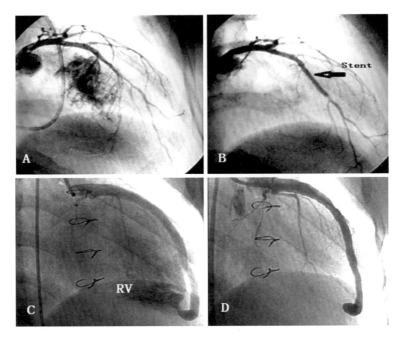

Figure 10-39   Pre- and post-TCC of LAD-PA fistula with a covered stent (A & B) and LAD-RV fistula with detachable balloon (C & D).

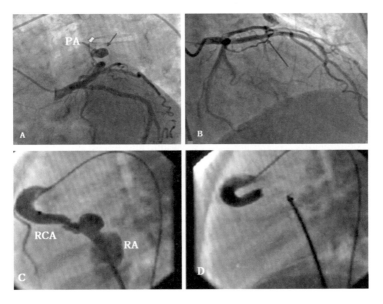

Figure 10-40   Pre- and post-TCC of LAD-PA fistula (A & B) and RCA-RA fistula (C & D) with coils.

287

Common complications:

—Arrhythmia;

—Coronary artery spasm (especially distal coronary artery);

—Coronary artery dissection;

—Residual shunt, hemolysis and hemoglobinuria after operation;

—Falling off, displacement and ectopic embolism of occluder;

—Valve damage;

—IE;

—Emergent thoracotomy is required;

—Peripheral vascular complications.

Sometimes, the treatment schemes and strategies for CAP are similar to CAF (Table 10-5), and the instruments are also the same (Figures, 10-41, 10-42, 10-43, and 10-44). The common therapeutic instruments for CAP include PTFE covered stent, microspheres, coils, and gelatin sponges. The small perforated vessel and the distal coronary artery are not suitable for

Table 10-5 Key Principles on the Indications and Techniques of CTO-PCI

1	The principal indication for CTO-PCI is to improve symptoms.
2	Dual ICA and thorough, structured angiographic review should be performed in every case.
3	Use of microcatheter is essential for guidewire support.
4	There are 4 CTO crossing strategies: antegrade wire escalation, antegrade dissection/reentry, retrograde wire escalation, and retrograde dissection/reentry.
5	Change of equipment and technique increases the likelihood of success and improves the efficiency of the procedure.
6	Centers and physicians performing CTO-PCI should have the necessary equipment, expertise, or experience to optimize success and minimize and manage complications.
7	Every effort should be made to optimize stent deployment in CTO-PCI, including the frequent use of intravascular imaging.

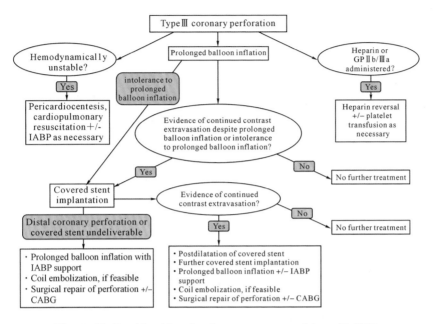

Figure 10-41 Algorithm for the management of type Ⅲ CAP.

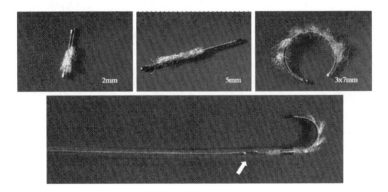

Figure 10-42 Tracker-10 spring coil (Boston). Platinum polyester fiber coil, compatible with 0.014 guidewire, which could be used as its pusher (arrow).

placement of covered stent. Among them, spring coil and microspheres are especially suitable for those needle-like CAP. Japanese doctors once injected a small piece of adipose tissue into the perforation site of the distal vessel through a microcatheter (before injection, and the adipose tissue was infiltrated in the contrast agent to facilitate accurate positioning). Its effect is

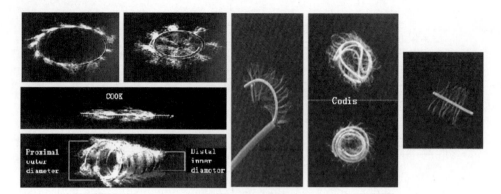

Figure 10-43　Platinum synthetic fiber spring coils (Cook and Codis).

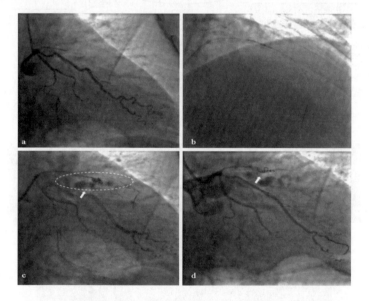

Figure 10-44　Tracker-10 spring coil (Boston) for treatment of LAD perforation.
a: The proximal LAD and middle LCX were totally occluded, and the formation of
the lateral branches was seen; b: The crosswire NT guidewire passed through the
occlusion lesion of LAD to reach the distal end, and balloon (1.5 mm × 20 mm) 6
atm dilated; c: Ellis type Ⅲ perforation (arrow), and the contrast agent flowed to
the pericardial cavity; d: An attempt was made to seal LAD with a balloon to heal
the perforation, but it was ineffective, so the tracker-10 spring coil was sent to the
perforation through the rapid transit microcatheter, and the contrast agent leakage
of LAD disappeared. At 1 hour, 12 hours, and 24 hours after operation and follow-
up before discharge, Echo showed a small amount of pericardial effusion without
pericardial tamponade.

similar to the spring coil, and the adipose tissue can be completely absorbed after the perforation healing.

Section II   Surgery

CAF is uncommon, and its treatments include percutaneous and surgical revascularization, both of which are associated with technical challenges. Furthermore, surgical intervention is a preferred treatment for giant CAF, including AN resection, bypassing when necessary, and closure of CAF (Figure 10-45).

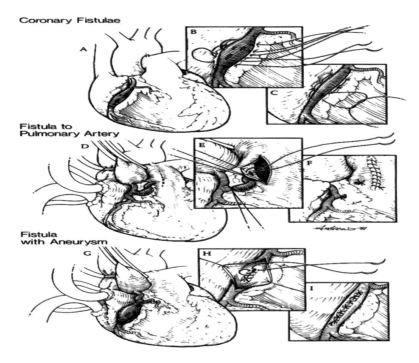

Figure 10-45   Technical types of surgical treatment of CAF.

Kitahara H reported a 39-year-old man with CAPF ligation and mitral valve repair through a mini-thoracotomy approach (Figure 10-46).

Surgical treatment was once considered the only feasible treatment (Figures 10-47, 10-48). From decades of surgical practice, the surgical effect

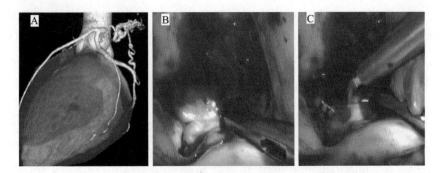

Figure 10-46 A: 3-D reconstruction indicated CAPF; Thoracoscopic view, CAPF was seen on the roof of LA (B) and occluded with metal clips (C).

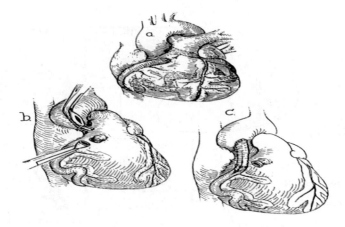

Figure 10-47 Schematic diagram of surgical operation of LCA-RV fistula in 1963.

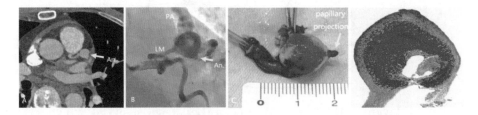

Figure 10-48 A: CT findings showed a 1.5-cm-diameter AN (arrow) derived from LM; B: ICA showed AN with a papillary projection (arrow) and shunt flow of the coronary artery to PA; C: The AN with a papillary projection (arrow) was surgically remove; D: Histological findings. Masson's trichrome stain (×40) showed that the internal elastic membrane had disappeared at the papillary projection.

of CAF is good, but the patients have a risk during and after the operation. The operative mortality is about 2%, the incidence of post-operative AMI is 3%–6%, and 4% of the patients have recurrence and recanalization of CAF. After long-term follow-up, most of the patients' clinical symptoms disappeared, and their cardiac function returned to normal.

For asymptomatic infant patients, the operation can be delayed; patients with small shunt flow, Qp/Qs below 1.3, and elderly asymptomatic CAF may not undergo surgery. However, for patients with critical symptoms and large shunt flow, active treatment should be recommended. Wood J reported the surgical treatment for a newborn patient with giant CAF (Figure 10-49).

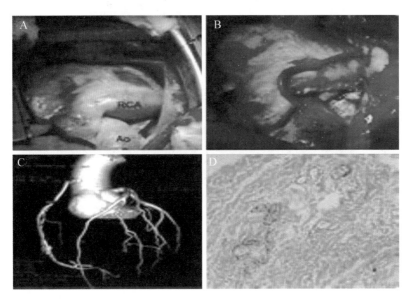

Figure 10-49   CT image, surgical fields and histological finding of RCA-LV fistula.

Many scholars have reported the single-center studies of surgical treatment of CAF. A large number of clinical experiences showed that the success rate of surgery was high, the complications were few, and the incidence of the residual shunt was lower than that of TCC (Figures 10-50, 10-51, and 10-52).

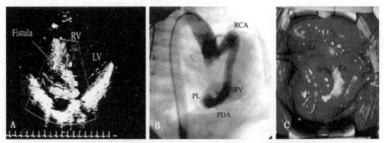

Figure 10-50   Echo, angiogram and surgical field of RCA-RV fistula.

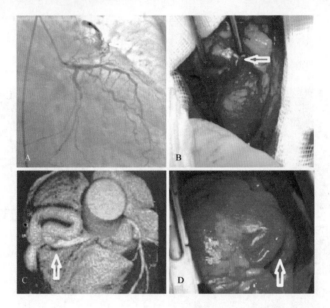

Figure 10-51   A & B: Angiogram and surgical field of LAD-PA fistula;   C & D: CT image and surgical field of CAF with AN.

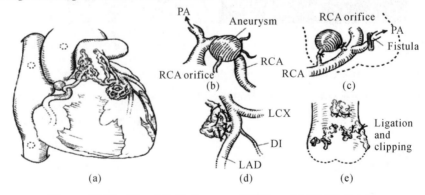

Figure 10-52   Visual field diagram of RCA and LAD-PA fistula.

In addition, the patients with CAF and AN should be treated as early as possible. The reasons are as followings: (a) The large AN compresses the myocardial cavity or distal coronary artery and causes myocardial ischemia, and then the heart gradually expands and even causes CHF; (b) If thrombosis occurs in AN, thrombus shedding can lead to coronary embolism and AMI.

Surgery is usually performed under general anesthesia, and continuous monitoring of ECG is required during the operation to determine whether there is myocardial ischemia. TEE is better for intraoperation monitoring, which can not only observe whether there is an abnormal movement of ventricular wall, but also determine the residual shunt. It has been reported that Starfish heart positioner was used in surgical treatment to ensure the stability of coronary blood flow supply during surgery (Figure 10-53).

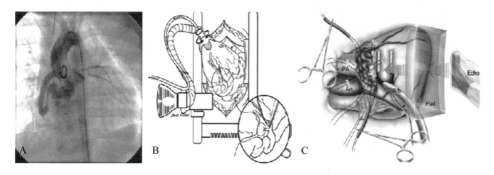

Figure 10-53   Application of cardiac locator and TEE in CAF surgery.

This device can reduce the chance of directly touching the patient's heart, thus lightening the pressure on the coronary artery and better exposing the surgical field. Common surgical methods include ligation or severing and suture at the end of the main branch, extra-arterial or tangential suture, transcardiac fistula closure or repair, and open CAF and repair (Figures 10-54, 10-55, and 10-56).

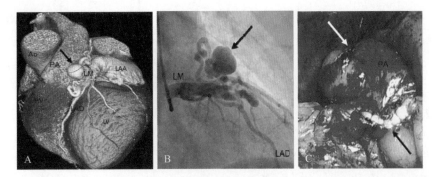

Figure 10-54 A & B: CTA and angiogram demonstrated a mesh-like network of arteries arising from LM and LAD with AN draining into PA; C: Intra-operative view showed AN with feeding vessel tied off (white arrow) and the oversewn PA (black arrow).

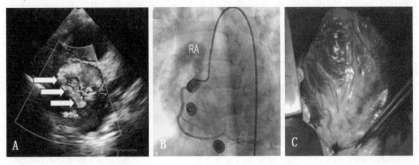

Figure 10-55 A & B: Echo and angiogram showed RCA-RA fistula; C: Surgical field.

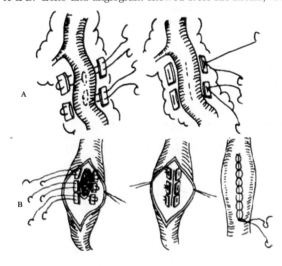

Figure 10-56 Suture and repair of lower tangent fistula (A); Open CAF and repair (B).

Surgical methods (Figure 10-57):

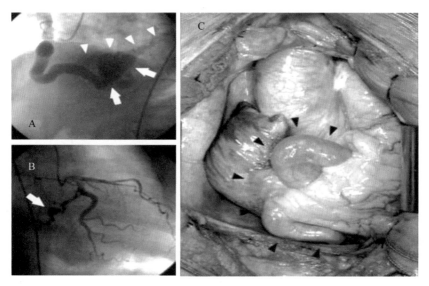

Figure 10-57   Angiograms and surgical field of multiple CAF. A: RCA-CS fistula;
B: Small CAF of LCX; C: Surgical field.

(1) Cut off ligation or tangential suture ligation without CPB. It has the advantages of simple operation, low operation cost, and good effect on patients with CAPF (Figure 10-58). The disadvantage is that the operative field is unclear and difficult to damage the coronary artery, affect the myocardial blood supply, and eventually lead to post-operative myocardial ischemia or AMI.

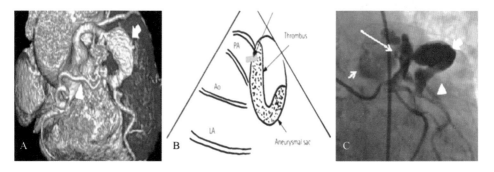

Figure 10-58   A & B: RCA-PA fistula and LAD aneurysm with thrombosis,
4.1 cm × 4.0 cm; C: Angiogram showed LAD-PA fistula with aneurysm.

(2) Operation under CPB: (a) Incision of coronary artery and direct suture or patch-repair for the patients with obvious expansion. This method has a clear visual field and accurate suture; (b) Intracardiac suture: It is better to use this method when the coronary expansion is unclear or the fistula enters the cavity from the back of the heart.

CPB support is unnecessary if the lesion is single and the anatomical relationship is clear, and only a simple ligation operation may be required. However, CPB is required in the following cases (Figures 10-59, 10-60):

(1) When the coronary artery is significantly expanded or combined with AN, the exact location of the fistula can not be determined from the heart surface, so it is necessary to open the coronary artery or perform coronary angioplasty at the same time.

(2) Fistula behind the heart, and difficult to expose the surgical field, such as RV inflow tract, CS, or posterior ventricular wall.

(3) The PA or cardiac cavity should be opened and repaired.

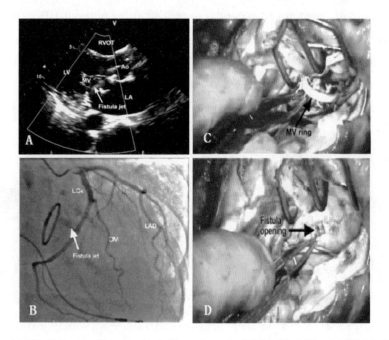

Figure 10-59　Echo, angiogram (A & B) and surgical field (C & D) of LCX-LA fistula.

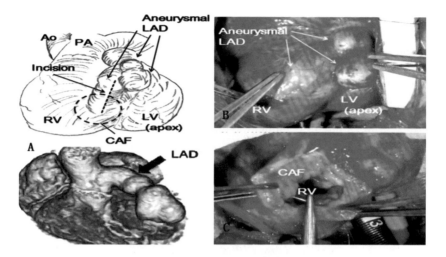

Figure 10-60   A: CTA and diagram of LAD-RV fistula with 10mm dilated LAD and AN; B & C: operation field.

（4）Patients with other CHD or CAA need surgical correction at the same time, such as AN incision or resection, thrombus removal, valve replacement, and CABG.

Post-operative complications:

a. Residual shunt;

b. Myocardial ischemia, ST segment changes or AMI;

c. Arrhythmia;

d. Sustained expansion of the coronary artery, and the twisted coronary artery has long-term stenosis and occlusion;

e. Stroke.

Among these, residual fistula and myocardial ischemia are the most common complications, with an early incidence of 4% and 3.7%, respectively. In recent years, the incidence of these familiar problems has been significantly diminished after mattress sutures or patch repairs. If the complications mentioned above occur, intra-operative TEE and ECG can be used to determine the diagnosis, and the appropriate treatment can be performed.

The incidence of complications is related to age. The mortality and the incidence of complications underwent surgery were 1% and 7% before the age of 20, 7% and 23% after the age of 20, respectively. Recent studies have shown that the safety of the operation is significantly improved, and the mortality of CAF without other CHD is less than 1%. A large number of reports at home and abroad indicate that most of the patients receiving surgical treatment have no clinical symptoms in the follow-up several years. Still, more detailed follow-up reports (including Echo and angiographic review) suggested that 10% of the patients have a residual shunt. Jeong EH analyzed the imaging changes before and after the operation of CAF with AN (Figure 10-61)

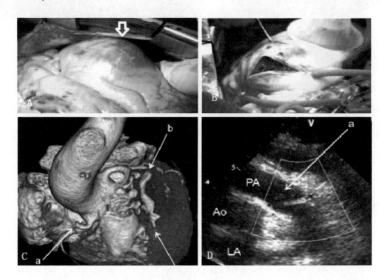

Figure 10-61 Surgical field of AN and post-operative Echo and CT image.
A: Tumor cavity with thrombus; B: PA incision; C: Coronary artery and AN ligation site; D: Residual shunt.

Spunda R reported a 70-year-old woman with a rare combination of AN associated with CAF, which drained into PA. The patient was treated surgically because of the symptomatic course of the disease (Figure 10-62).

Peng Y reported a 37-year-old man with 2-year history of chest pain that frequently occurred during moderate exercise. CTA and TTE, TEE showed dilated tortuous RCA and enlarged CS with a bright flow. Angiogram

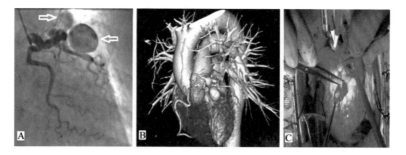

Figure 10-62   A: Angiogram showed 2 AN. The cranial and smaller AN was supplied by vessels that originated from the left and right coronary arteries; B: CTA showed the position of both AN and their supplying arteries; C: Peri-operative photograph of removal of adhering thrombus in AN.

confirmed the hairpin-like RCA-CS fistula, which was difficult to plug. The patient made a rapid recovery after the operation, and had no chest pain during exercise at 3-month follow-up (Figure 10-63).

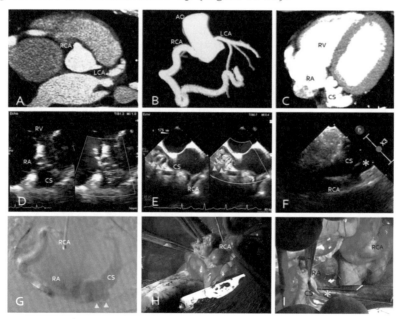

Figure 10-63   A-C: CTA showed the origin of tortuous dilated RCA, its course and dilated CS; D-F: TTE and TEE showed a blood flow from the dilated CS, and hairpin-like CAF (arrow, asterisk); G. Angiogram demonstrated the termination of RCA fistula (arrow); H-I: At surgery, the tortuous dilated RCA could be seen, while the defect was corrected in CS (asterisk).

Liu H described a novel technique of MIS for CAP patients without CPB via parasternal mini-thoracotomy. This technique has been proven safe and effective and may be useful for patients with CAPF (Figure 10-64). Up to now, MIS has been used more frequently for cardiac diseases. Current data has demonstrated that MIS provides several advantages for patients compared with conventional cardiac surgery. However, as we all know, the MIS has rarely been used in CAF.

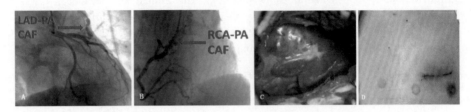

Figure 10-64 A & B: Angiogram showed LAD-PA fistula and RCA-PA fistula; C: Operative field of CAPF; D: Skin incision.

Psychological nursing should be accomplished well before the operation. Bedside ECG should be done every day to observe whether there is myocardial ischemia, diminish the patient's vigorous activities, reduce myocardial oxygen consumption, and avoid peri-operative AMI. The key points of nursing are to closely monitor heart rhythm and heart rate, improve electrolyte balance and cardiac function, and prevent secondary thrombosis.

Chapter XI Complications and prognosis

Highlights

- Once diagnosed, CAF should be treated surgically. With the increase of age, the patients have more complications, including CHF, IE, AMI or fistula rupture, the sudden death of unknown origins and others.
- The evolution of the natural course of CAF is uncertain, and natural closure and spontaneous rupture are extremely rare.
- If the fistula is small and the patient has no symptoms, follow-up observation can be carried out without other special treatment. Patients undergoing surgery or TCC also need routine and regular Echo examinations.

Although the prognosis of CAF have large differences, the possible complications of patients in the future will be the ultimate determinant. In adults with stable hemodynamics, some patients may be asymptomatic for life. For other patients with complications such as CHF, atrial/ventricular arrhythmia, and pericardial tamponade, it is necessary to immediately improve the complications and then treat CAF by TCC or surgery. Although the recurrence of CAF is rare, surgery can decrease the recanalization compared with TCC.

Spontaneous closure of congenital CAF is rare, and IE and other complications can occur in 5%–10% of patients of any age, but regular or routine IE prophylaxis is no longer recommended. The natural history of congenital CAF has a long and slow progress in size over many years, but the progressive enlargement and spontaneous rupture are rare. Rupture generally occurs due to aneurysmal dilation, coronary wall weakening, and atherosclerotic plaque. Small CAF can occasionally close naturally, and its mechanism may be thromboembolic closure of blood vessels, and fibrosis surrounding the fistula.

The risk of IE was calculated to be 0.25% per patient-year. Possible complications of CAF are dilatation of the coronary artery, mural thrombosis, rupture, atherosclerotic deposition, aneurysm formation, calcification, intimal ulceration, intimal rupture, medial degeneration, side-branch obstruction. The exact percentage of spontaneous closure of CAF remains unknown but relatively rare. A review of the literature showed that fistula draining into RV had some chances to close spontaneously. Thrombus within the fistula is rare and may cause spontaneous closure, but also induce AMI, and atrial or ventricular arrhythmia.

The small fistula can exist continuously without any changes; the fistula of moderate size can gradually increase, but the progress is slow, and it often takes more than 15 years; the patients with huge fistula may present with shortness of breath, CHF and angina pectoris in infancy or after entering the youth. Because the fistula in most cases is generally small, the clinical symptoms of volume overload only appear after age 50.

Patients with CAF who underwent percutaneous or surgical closure have a good prognosis. Life expectancy is normal, with recurrence rate ranging from 9 to 19% for TCC and 25% for surgical ligation. It is worth noting that the risk of developing atherosclerosis is increased with CAF and abnormal ectasia of coronary arteries.

Clinical follow-up with Echo 1 month after percutaneous or surgical CAF closure is recommended. If the patient remains asymptomatic and Echo shows improved results, a close follow-up with Echo evaluation every 6-12 months should be pursued initially and then every 2-3 years.

Section I Complications

On the whole, complications of CAF, such as left-right shunt, CHF, AMI, pericardial effusion, aneurysm formation and rupture, hemopericardium, pulmonary hypertension, IE, syncope, stroke, and sudden death, may occur with low incidence.

(1) IE

Untreated congenital CAF may be associated with serious complications (Table 11-1), such as IE, which is considered more dangerous than CAF itself. Although CAF occurs more frequently in RCA (50%–60%) and the fistula most often enters PA, RV, and RA (80%), complications involving IE are rare. CAF in adult subjects complicated by IE, affecting both the right and left cardiac valves with valvular destruction and perforation has been reported. IE has also been reported in children with CCF.

Table 11-1   Possible complications of CAF

Complications	Features
Cardiovascular	Myocardial infarction, stroke, aneurysm, and rupture
Pulmonary vascular	Pulmonary hypertension
Infections	Bacterial endocardrtis, septic pulmonary embolism, and septic renal embolism
Valvular	Incompetence, dysfunction, and perforation
Pericardial	Hemopericardium, pericardial effusion, and tamponade
Myocardial	Congestive heart failure
Arrhythmia	Supraventricular arrhythmia, ventricular arrhythmia, and sudden death

In 1973, Liberthson RR reported 13 cases of CAF and reviewed the clinical history of 174 cases previously reported in the literature. In 1981, Lowe JE reported 28 patients with CAF identified at Duke Medical Center between 1960 and 1981. The authors state that IE is a common symptom. However, these authors recommend that "nearly all patients with major CAF be considered for surgical correction" due to the eventual development of either "CHF, angina pectoris, AMI, IE, aneurysm formation with rupture or embolization, or the development of pulmonary hypertension". In 2013, Ahn DS reported a case of RCA-LV fistula associated with IE of the mitral valve.

The patient, a 27-year-old man, presented for mitral repair 2 months after being diagnosed with Streptococcus viridans IE. Diagnosis of aneurysmal RCA with fistulous drainage into LV at the base of the posterior mitral leaflet was made by TEE and confirmed at surgery. Ong ML in 1993 reported a 17-year-old female with congenital RCA-CS fistula presented with recurrent septic pulmonary embolism secondary to tricuspid valve endocarditis (Figure 11-1).

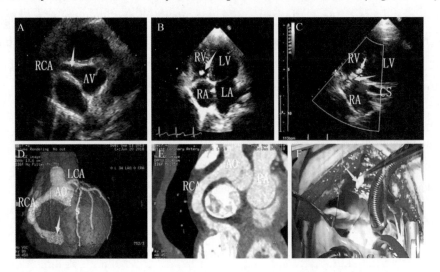

Figure 11-1 TTE showed the dilated RCA (A, arrow) and vegetation (B, arrow); C: CDE showed abnormal turbulent flow (large arrow) and vegetation (small arrow); D-F: MDCT images showed the whole dilated journey of RCA and several fistulas (arrows); F: Vegetation in operative field (arrow).

IE may occur not only in patients with CCF but also in patients with CAVF. Similarly, IE is not only reported in congenital CAF but also in acquired CAF. At the beginning of the last century, vegetation complicating IE was reported in pediatric postmortem cases of CCF. Nowadays, antemortem diagnosis is easily established due to the increased awareness and widespread and early use of noninvasive diagnostic modalities.

The estimated incidence of IE has been reported to occur from 3% to 12% of cases. The risk of IE was calculated to be 0.25%–0.4% per patient-year. In 1992, Fernandes ED found that IE developed in association with CCF in 1 out of the 93 patients. On the other hand, in 2015, Kaminska M identified 18 reports of patients with CAF complicated with IE in the period from 2000 to 2015. IE may be an initial manifestation of CAF or may develop during the course of disease; IE may occur in isolated CAF or complex CAF associated with other CHD.

Accordingly, in the current review, fever was the most common symptom in 60% of subjects, followed by fatigue and sepsis. In 2006, upon reviewing the worldwide literature, IE was reported in 2% of pediatric subjects. The subacute presentation of bacterial endocarditis has been reported in both pediatric subjects with CCF and adult patients with CAVF. In 1984, Slater J reported recurrent IE in a middle-aged man with CCF. The most common microorganisms causing IE include: Streptococci, S. aureus, Enterococcus species, HACEK organisms, and fungi. The rate of subsequent bacteremia (Streptococcus species) following TEE is estimated at 0%–25% and 30%–100% after dental extractions.

In the current review, the most common pathogenic bacteria of IE are Streptococci (50%) and Staphylococci (30%). Tsai WC reported that the dental procedure could induce the occurrence of IE, and Staphylococci have been detected in a few cases. However, Streptococcus species are the most commonly isolated microorganisms from blood cultures. In patients with CAF complicated with IE, valvular and nonvalvular involvement has been reported. IE was associated with nonvalvular vegetations protruding at the drainage site of RV (Figure 11-2).

Small or large nonvalvular vegetation, as well as valvular vegetation located in the atrioventricular valves or semilunar valves, have been observed. Earlier reports have indicated that congenital CCF is more prone to the development of IE than CAVF. The reason for this is that the high-speed jet lesion may cause damage to the endothelium, leading to local vulnerable nidus near the drainage site of the fistula. Furthermore, it is assumed that vegetation and perforation occur because of the increased and abnormal turbulent flow.

(2) Septic embolization

Septic emboli to the lungs and kidneys were reported in 6/25 (24%) of

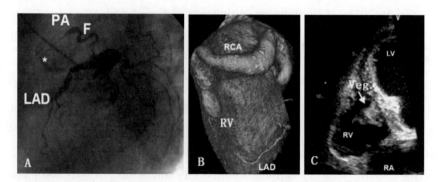

Figure 11-2 A: Fistulous jet (*) of CAF (F) arising from LAD and terminating into PA might cause lesion of the endothelial wall and act as a nidus (*); B: MDCT showed RCA-RV fistula; C: An oscillating echogenic mass attached to RV inferoseptal wall (arrow).

the reviewed subjects. The majority of the septic pulmonary emboli were caused by S. aureus (80%). Dilatation and AN formation of the vessels were present in 5 of them. Termination was coronary-cameral in 4 and coronary-vascular in 2 of the subjects. These findings emphasize that aggressive pharmacological and nonpharmacological treatment strategies are recommended to prevent such complications (Figure 11-3).

It is clear and definite that jet-related intimal lesions at the drainage site of CAF may be the site of endocarditis. In the case of right-sided origin of CAF with left-sided endocarditis, infectious emboli may migrate via the pulmonary circulation to the left-sided cardiac valves. Left-sided valvular endocarditis caused by septic pulmonary thrombus has been reported in a few CAF cases with right-sided origin. Some authors declared that it was unclear which was the first focus of infection, the CAF itself or the infected valve lesion.

In the current review, the applied treatment modalities include intravenous antibiotics, surgical ligation of the fistula with or without CABG, valve repair, and single or multiple valve replacement. Surgical closure of the fistula was frequently performed (64%), after completing effective antibiotic treatment, but pulmonary thromboembolism (PTE) was successfully improved in some selected cases (8%). A prior course of intravenous

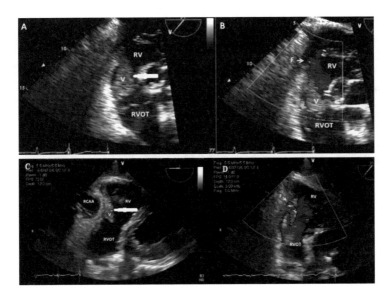

Figure 11-3   A: TEE showed a vegetation (V) in RVOT; B: Attachment was by
stalk to RV free wall at site of the fistula drainage; C: Vegetation attached to RV
free wall after therapy; D: TEE showed color flow signal in RV near RVOT
consistent with fistulous drainage from AN.

antibiotics with a variable length, from days to months was reported in the
literature. However, the time between diagnosis and intervention was
documented in a limited number of the reviewed reports.

Spontaneous closure of the fistula (4%) has occurred via the formation
of thrombus following an episode of IE. Spontaneous closure, not associated
with IE, has been observed in pediatric and adult subjects caused by
atherosclerotic and thrombotic changes.

It is widely accepted that the onset of symptoms including typical or
atypical chest pain, dyspnea, or palpitation due to left-right shunt may occur
with Qp/Qs > 1.5. It should be emphasized that antibiotic prophylaxis is
strongly advised for pediatric and adult patients with congenital CAF.

(3) CAF related symptoms

Han JS reported 1 case with LM-RA fistula causing acute cardiac failure
and arrest (Figure 11-4). Shimada S reported 1 case with CHF and
myocardial ischemia in neonates with CAF (Figure 11-5).

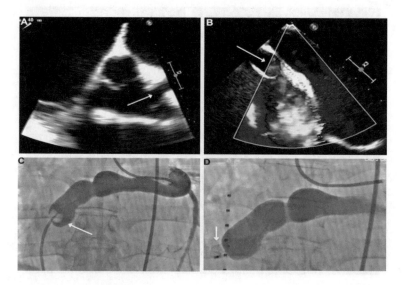

Figure 11-4　A-B: TEE demonstrated enlarged LM (arrow) and the severely dilated RA with flow from the fistula (arrow); C-D: ICA demonstrated the filling of fistula with contrast agent. The fistula was occluded distally from RA by balloon catheter inserted using venous approach (arrow).

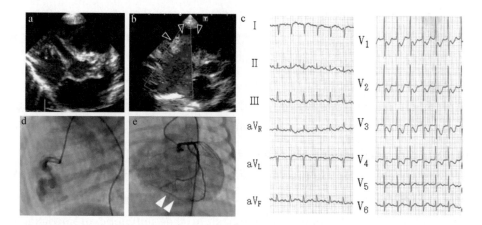

Figure 11-5　a: Echo on the first day of age showed a markedly enlarged RCA; b: CDE showed CAF (open arrows) draining into RV; c: ECG at 7 days of age showed significant ST depression in lead V1-V4; d: Angiograms of RCA showed significantly dilated RCA draining into RV; e: Collateral arteries (white arrows) from LCA to the distal RCA.

Chen P described a case of SVCS, which was secondary to the compression by huge AN formed in recurrent CAF, as a long-term complication associated with surgical treatment (Figure 11-6).

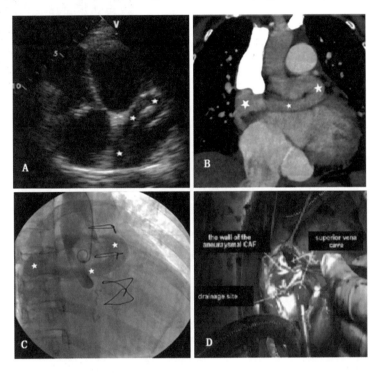

Figure 11-6　A: Echo revealed the ostium of the dilated LM and the fistula originated from LM, coursing around the aorta (stars); B & C: MDCT and angiogram confirmed the presence of recurrent fistula (stars) and the grossly aneurysmal dilation of the fistula compressing SVC (stars); D: Surgical field.

Battisha A reported a 67-year-old female with no modifiable cardiovascular risk factors who had an unwitnessed sudden death at home during her ongoing evaluation of CAF detected incidentally between LAD and PA (Figure 11-7).

Regarding sudden cardiac death, Lau G reported a 29-year-old male with a history of unknown congenital cardiovascular disease, for which no surgery was performed. This man collapsed suddenly at home, and then transferred to the emergency room, where resuscitation attempts were unsuccessful. On autopsy, the cause of death was myocardial ischemia related to right-sided

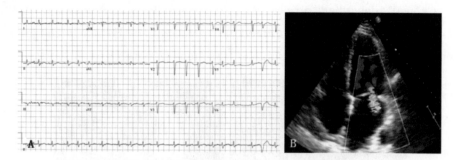

Figure 11-7　A: ECG demonstrated atrial fibrillation with episode of premature ventricular contractions; B: TEE revealed LVEF of 25% to 30% with severe global hypokinesis with regional variation, diastolic function was not assessed due to atrial fibrillation. It showed also mitral and tricuspid regurgitation.

fistula, in which the RCA was involved, along with LV hypertrophy.

Meric M described an extensive fistula complicated with fatal ventricular arrhythmia due to ischemia and LV dysfunction. A cardioverter defibrillator was implanted to prevent sudden cardiac death (Figure 11-8).

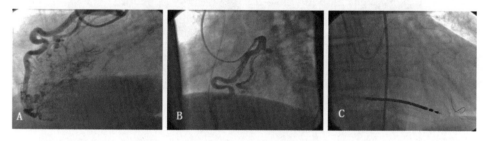

Figure 11-8　A: Angiogram before intervention showed LAD-LV fistula; B: Implantation of coil via microcatheter to the distal LAD; C: ICD implanted.

Wu DF reported a case clinically diagnosed as Wellens syndrome by ECG findings, which was a pre-infarction stage of severe stenosis or occlusion of the proximal LAD and might lead to extensive anterior wall AMI without timely intervention. ICA subsequently showed the fistula originating from LAD and draining into PA. The ECG findings then returned to normal after the fistula had been closed by controlled-release coils (Figure 10-9, 10-10).

Erdogan E described a rare case of RCA fistula draining to RA, manifesting in chest pain and pulmonary hypertension. The fistula was

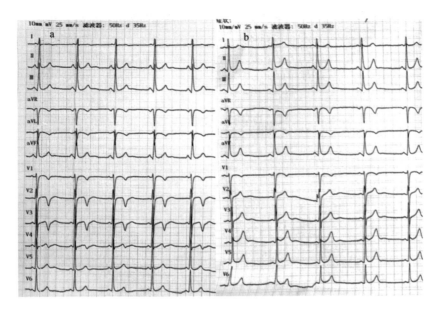

Figure 11-9   a: ECG at presentation with deep symmetric T-wave inversion in lead V1-V3, and biphasic T-wave was present in lead V4; b: ECG after the intervention showed sinus rhythm and improved T-wave inversion in the anteroseptal leads.

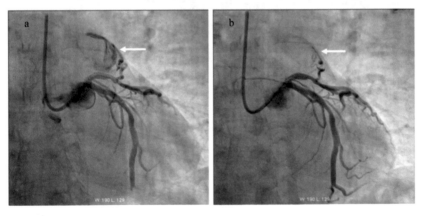

Figure 11-10   a: Angiogram showed the fistula originating from LAD and draining into PA; b: The fistula had been closed by controlled-release coils.

detected on TEE during the workup for pulmonary hypertension (Figures 11-11, 11-12).

Lahiri S reported a case of coronary thrombosis and AMI in a child following device closure of CAF. After a clear understanding of CCF, risk

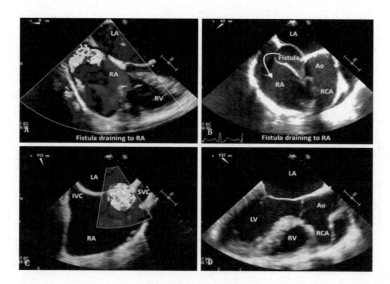

Figure 11-11   A: Coronary fistula draining to RA close to the posterior interatrial septum; B: Dilated proximal RCA, and draining to RA (white arrow); C: Adjacent to interatrial septum, close to SVC, fistula's ostium was seen with 3 cm × 2.2 cm in diameter; D: Dilated proximal RCA was seen.

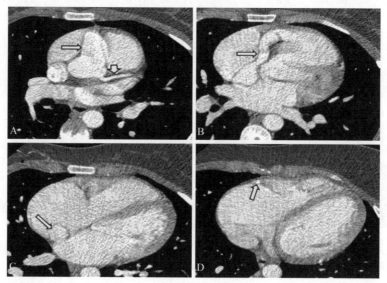

Figure 11-12   A: The markedly dilated proximal RCA (arrow) had a diameter of 21 mm. LM (arrowhead) was normal; B: The dilated tortuous sinoatrial nodal branch (arrow) travelled along the interatrial septum; C: The fistula orifice (arrow) opened to RA through the posterosuperior of the interatrial septum; D: RCA (arrow) followed its normal diameter after giving the sinoatrial branch.

factors for thrombosis and post-closure sequela, the aggressive anticoagulant is imperative for the treatment of coronary events following CAF closure (Figures 10-13, 10-14).

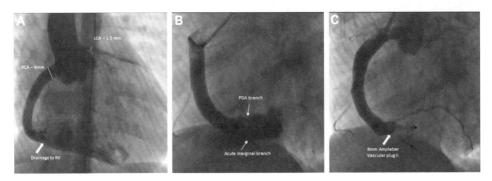

Figure 11-13   Angiogram demonstrated large distal RCA fistula draining to RV (A, arrow), and distal PDA branches (B, arrows), underwent successful closure using Amplatzer vascular plug Ⅱ (C).

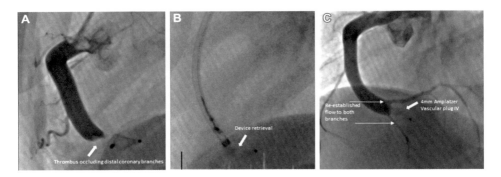

Figure 11-14   Angiogram demonstrated RCA thrombosis occluding the distal coronary branches following device closure (A), treated by thrombolysis and device retrieval (B) and new Amplatzer vascular plug Ⅳ placement (C).

Shrestha BK reported a case of coronary artery-CS fistula with coil migration into RA after percutaneous closure and required surgical intervention (Figure 11-15).

Neerod KJ presented a 26-year-old male patient with symptoms of chest pain and dyspnea. He was diagnosed with RCA-LA fistula and AN. The closure of the fistula was done using an autologous pericardial patch under CPB (Figures 10-16, 10-17).

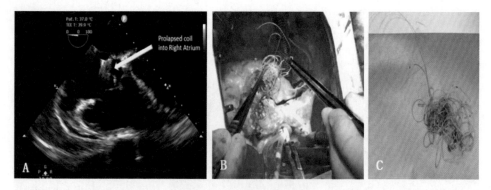

Figure 11-15 A: Migrated (prolapsed) coil into RA; B: Removal of migrated coil via right atriotomy; C: Removal of coil.

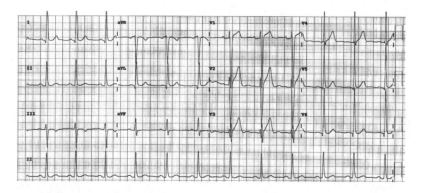

Figure 1-16 ECG showed ST changes in the anterior leads and evidence of LV enlargement.

Bessho S successfully treated a patient who presented with cardiac tamponade due to ruptured CAPF. Taha ME reported the case of a 68-year-old woman with a family history of premature cardiac diseases who presented with ischemic chest pain and elevated troponin levels. Her ECG and troponin were suggestive of NSTEMI, for which she was initially treated medically and later underwent ICA. Unexpectedly, ICA revealed patent coronary arteries, and the authors discovered evidence of coronary artery-LV fistula in addition to angiographic evidence of Takotsubo cardiomyopathy. A working diagnosis of Takotsubo cardiomyopathy was made, for which she was treated medically with the improvement of symptoms and later in the imaging

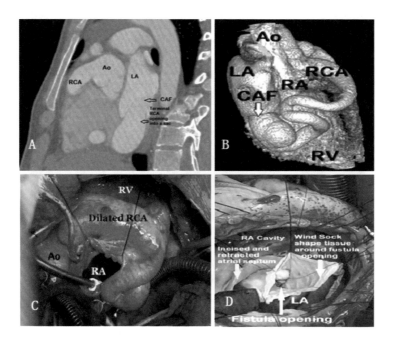

Figure 1-17   A & B: CTA showed origin of the dilated coronary artery from the ascending aorta, and tortuous RCA-LA fistula; C & D: Operative photograph showed fistula tract of the aneurysmal RCA and surrounding structures, and opening of the fistula tract of RCA into LA floor with a windsock guarding the orifice of the fistula.

findings (Figures 11-18, 11-19).

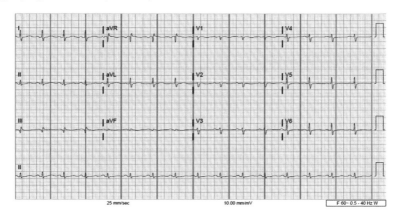

Figure 11-18   ECG showed poor R wave progression and borderline T wave changes.

317

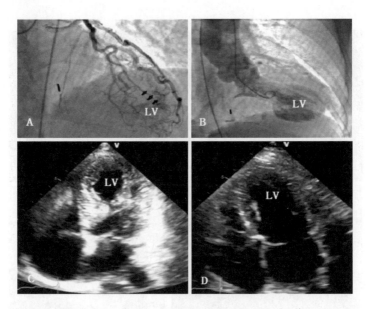

Figure 11-19   A: Angiogram showed fistula originating from LAD and draining into LV; B: Ventriculogram showed regional wall motion abnormality with apical ballooning of LV, a typical feature in Takotsubo; C: TTE demonstrated LVESV at the time of presentation. Pay attention to the apical ballooning and reduced function; D: TTE demonstrated LVESV at 4 weeks after discharge as a follow-up. Pay attention to the improvement in systolic function.

Pongbangli N reported a rare case of congenital CAF originating from LAD and terminating into PA. The patient presented with acute cardiac tamponade due to the rupture of large AN after being gored by a buffalo (Figure 11-20).

The case of a young woman with RCA-CS fistula was reported, and she had dilated coronary artery causing ACS due to thrombogenesis in the puerperal period (Figure 11-21).

Ono R reported a 52-year-old woman who presented with dyspnea on exertion. Her ECG revealed an advanced atrioventricular block and left bundle branch block. CT scan confirmed 2 fistulas, from the conus branch of RCA and LAD into PA. The patient underwent pacemaker implantation (Figures 11-22, 11-23).

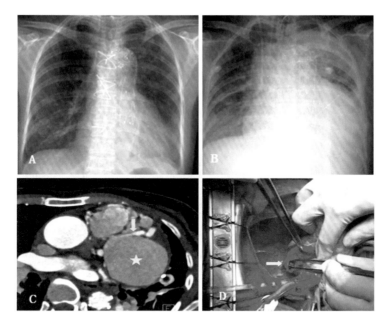

Figure 11-20   A: Chest X-ray on 3 days after thoracic endovascular AN repair (TEVAR); B: 7 days after TEVAR showed the increased cardiothoracic ratio suggesting the presence of pericardial effusion; C: Giant AN (asterisk) arising from LAD (arrow); D: Intra-operative findings demonstrated the rupture site of AN (arrow).

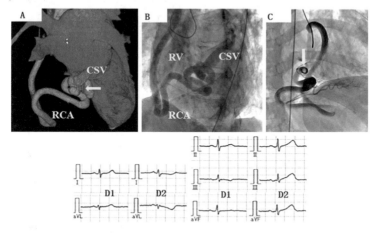

Figure 11-21   Cardiac images of the patient at 33 years of age. A & B: CT image and angiogram showed RCA-CS fistula and tortuous RCA. The junction of the RCA-CS was narrow (yellow arrow); C: Angiogram showed stagnant coronary flow and thrombogenesis in RCA-CS fistula (yellow arrow); D1: ECG before the delivery and D2 in emergency room, ST segment elevation in lead Ⅱ, Ⅲ, and aVF, and reciprocal ST depression in lead Ⅰ and aVL was observed.

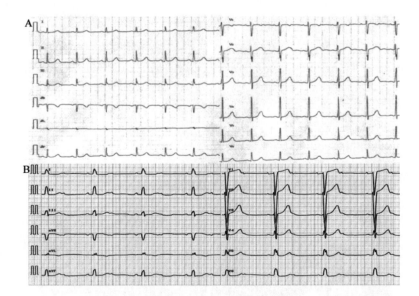

Figure 11-22 A: ECG 1 year before the current presentation showed normal sinus rhythm without bundle branch block; B: Present ECG showed advanced atrioventricular block (2:1 block) and new LBBB.

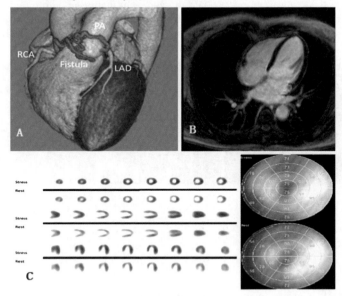

Figure 11-23 A: CT image showed the fistula from the conus branch of RCA and LAD draining into PA. The fistulas were highlighted in purple color; B: Late gadolinium enhancement was not detected in LV myocardium on CMR; C: Exercise myocardial perfusion SPECT demonstrated normal 99mTc-sestamibi uptake at stress and at rest.

Lee SH also reported a case presented with dilated cardiomyopathy, due to a large amount of shunt by CAF originating from a single coronary artery and draining into LV, and successfully treated with surgical ligation. TTE showed severe diffuse hypokinesia of LV with EF of 15%–20% (Figure 11-24).

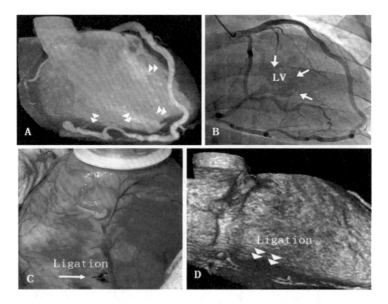

Figure 11-24   A & B: CT image and angiogram demonstrated direct drainage of LAD into LV (white arrows); C: The intra-operative image showed the enlarged and tortuous LAD was dissected near the base of LV and double ligation was done (white arrow); D: CT post-operative showed successful ligation of the distal PDA close to LV drainage site (white double arrowheads).

Section II   Prognosis

Small fistula is usually asymptomatic and has an excellent prognosis if managed medically with clinical and Echo follow-up every 2-5 years. In the case of symptomatic, large-sized, or giant fistula, an invasive treatment, by transcatheter approach or surgical ligation, is usually a reasonable choice, and both strategies show equivalent results at long-term follow-up. Antibiotic prophylaxis to prevent of IE is recommended in all CAF patients undergoing dental, gastrointestinal, or urological procedures. A life-long follow-up is always essential to ensure that the patients with CAF are not undergoing the progression of the disease or further cardiac complications.

Lee S reported a special case of spontaneous partial degenerative closure of CAF after drug treatment (Figure 11-25).

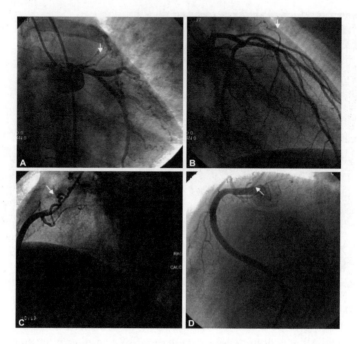

Figure 11-25 Angiographic changes of different outcomes of CAF. A & B: There was no significant change in reexamination of LCA-PA fistula after 2 years; C & D: RCA-PA fistula was partially closed 2 years later.

Schanzenbacher P reported a case of acquired RCA-RV fistula after AMI, which was later closed spontaneously (Figure 11-26).

Most patients with CAF successfully occluded by interventional treatment have a good prognosis. However, due to the possibility of recanalization, long-term follow-up of coronary artery expansion, thrombosis, calcification, and myocardial ischemia should be conducted. At the same time, the patients treated with conservative medical drugs should also be closely followed-up. McMahon CJ reported the results of a 3-year follow-up after coil closure (Figure 11-27).

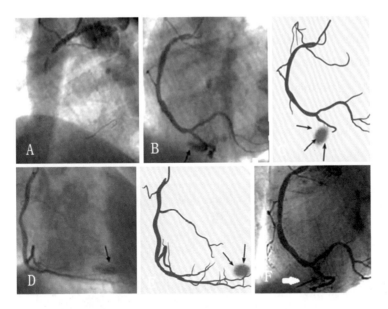

Figure 11-26   A: RCA total occlusion; B-E: Right posterior descending branch-RV fistula was found after stent implanted (C and E are diagrams); F: After 18 months of follow-up, it was found that CAF closed spontaneously.

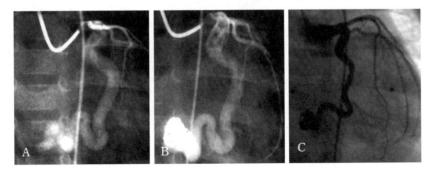

Figure 11-27   Angiograms before and after TCC. A: pre-operative CAF; B: Immediate angiogram after occlusion; C: Reexamination after 3 years.

Many scholars believe that a small amount of residual shunt can be reserved after interventional or surgical treatment of CAF, including the following effects: reduce the degree of blood stasis and prevent long-term intravascular thrombosis, stenosis, and myocardial ischemia. No special treatment is required for asymptomatic small CAF without localized tumor-like dilatation. After TCC, Aspirin and Clopidogrel or Ticagrelor should also be given for a long time (3-6 months). Statins have many effects such as lipid-lowering, anti-inflammatory, and anti-platelet aggregation. As a secondary prevention of CAD, statins may also have important benefits for atherosclerotic stenosis or thrombosis of CAF. Therefore, they should be given immediately after the operation.

Wang X reported a case of TCC of RCA-LV fistula with giant AN, and suggested that the progression of AN was a potential risk (Figure 11-28).

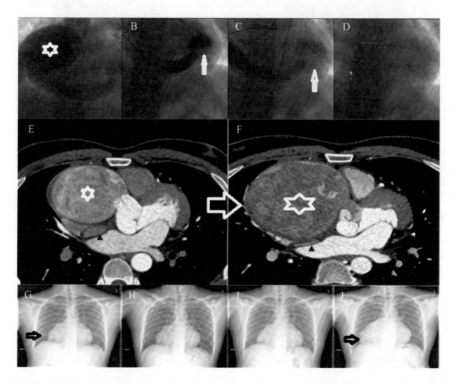

Figure 11-28 A-D: The distal diameter of the fistula was 4 mm, and TCC was performed successfully with Amplatzer duct occluder Ⅱ; E & F: During the follow-up of 2 years, the size of AN enlarged significantly; G-J: Increased cardiothoracic ratio (from 65% to 73%).

Yeung DF reported an unfortunate case of AN measuring 4.0 cm × 3.0 cm with fistula to PA, along with large pericardial effusion, which presumably resulted from its rupture (Figure 11-29).

Li X investigated long-term outcomes after CAF closure by following 79

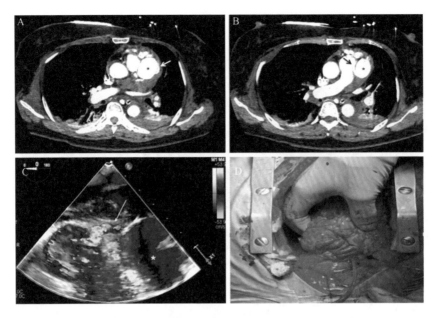

Figure 11-29   A: Large AN (black asterisk) with a fistulous connection originating from LAD (white arrow); B: Terminating in the main PA (black arrow); C: CDE highlighted its fistulous connection to PA originating from LCA (white arrow); D: Intra-operative view of LAD-PA fistula with AN.

patients for approximately 11 years. This research would help to improve our understanding of CAF and to identify the optimal surgical strategy for individual patients. The most common complication after CAF closure was thrombosis. Increased risk for thrombosis was associated with large fistula, distal-type CAF, and older age. Antiplatelet treatment did not appear to decrease the risk of thrombosis. The risk of thrombosis was lower among the patients with distal-type CAF treated with endocardial closure than those treated with epicardial ligation.

In conclusion, the long-term outcomes of CAF closure may not be as satisfactory as reported previously, and follow-up is of paramount importance. The surgical procedure should be individualized based on the size and classification of CAF. Given the very high incidence of thrombus formation, it is unclear whether antiplatelet therapy, systemic anticoagulation, or a combination of both will be the most effective in reducing post-operative thrombosis. Additional studies are necessary to elucidate the risks and benefits associated with CAF closure in adult and elderly patients (Figures 11-30, 11-31).

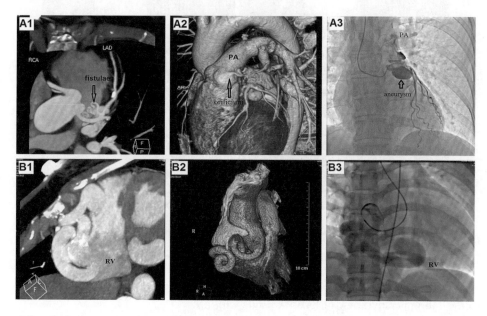

Figure 11-30　MDCT images (A1, A2, B1, B2) and angiograms (A3, B3) for various types of CAF. A1-A3: Proximal type. The CAF arose from the proximal segment of LAD and drained into PA. Tortuosity and AN formation of fistula vessel were observed. The entire LAD was of normal caliber; B1-B3: Distal type. The distal segment of RCA drained into RV. The entire RCA was severely dilated and tortuous.

Kim H evaluated the natural course of CAPF detected on CTA and proposed potential treatment strategies. Most CAPF identified on CTA have a favorable prognosis. Observation with optimal medical therapy (OMT) is usually an appropriate strategy, and fistula size is a possible determinant of surgical treatment.

Xiao Y evaluated the short- and medium-term efficacy, complications, and anticoagulant therapy related to TCC of CAF in children. TCC is feasible and safe in proximal and distal/medium-sized CAF patients. Post-operative anticoagulation with Aspirin or other drugs may prevent short- and medium-term thrombosis, but treatment course and safety need to be investigated for

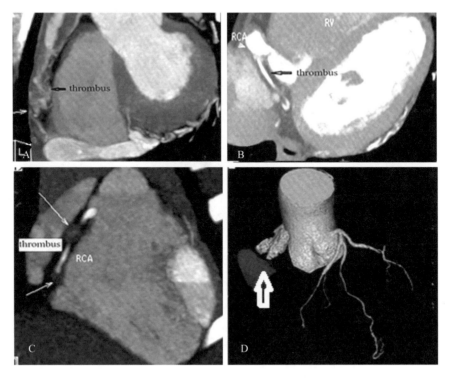

Figure 11-31   Follow-up of patients who had undergone CAF closure. A: Ring-shaped thrombus at the first crossing of RCA; B: Irregular parietal thrombus in RCA; C: The presence of a thrombus caused segmental occlusion in RCA; D: The entire RCA was completely occluded by the thrombus.

further follow-up (Figures 11-32, 11-33).

Christmann M retrospectively analyzed all patients with CAF diagnosed between 1993 and 2014 concerning treatment approaches and follow-up after closure. CAF in pediatric cardiology patients is an infrequent finding. Intervention in childhood is rarely needed; nevertheless, it is known that small fistulas may become relevant in adulthood. TCC techniques are effective and are considered the treatment of choice, especially in isolated CAF (Figure 11-34).

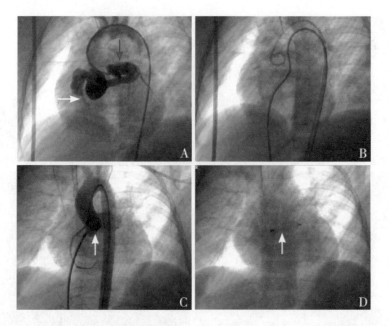

Figure 11-32   Female, 25 months old. A: Aortic angiogram showed LAD (red arrow) was tortuous, dilated and aneurysmal, and the fistula was located in RA (white); B: Establish arteriovenous orbit; C: The proximal end of the descending branch before plugging (arrow). There was no residual fistula after reexamination; D: The occluder (arrow) released the positive film.

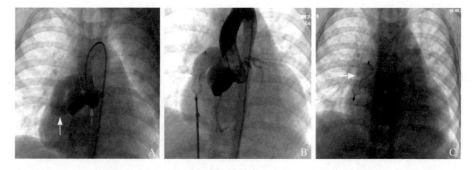

Figure 11-33   Female, 26 months old. A: Aortic angiogram showed dilated RCA (red arrow) and AN, and the fistula was located in RA (white arrow); B: Block the distal end of RCA (arrow). There was no residual fistula and the proximal branch was well developed; C: The occluder (arrow) released the positive film.

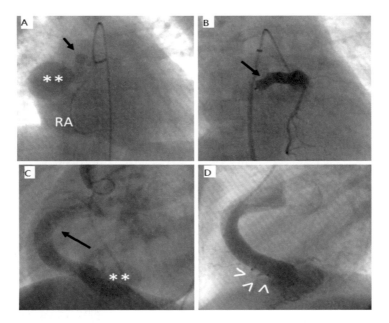

Figure 11-34   A: Angiogram showed CAF from RCA (arrow) connecting to RA via a large AN (∗∗); B: Completely closed CAF 45 min after implantation of Amplatzer vascular plug (arrow) in CAF; C: CAF (arrow) from RCA connecting to RV via an intracavitary AN (∗∗); D: Implantation of Amplatzer duct occluder Ⅱ in CAF.

Postscript

In 2015, under the guidance and help of Prof. Junbo Ge, an academician of the Chinese Academy of Sciences, we published the first monograph *Coronary Artery Fistula* in China, referring to more than 500 references before 2015. Over the past 8 years, cardiovascular technology has advanced by leaps and bounds, and a large number of papers on coronary artery fistula have been published. We reviewed and cited more than 300 relevant documents since 2015 and recompiled this book in English.

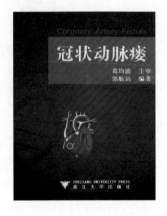

Here, we want to express our admiration and gratitude to the authors for their hard and excellent work.

When clinical medicine is approved as a national first-class undergraduate major, we would like to thank the post-graduate students and members of the scientific research team:

Longbin Liu, Fukang Xu, Yafei Shi, Haitao Lü, Zheng Ji, Xiaoya Zhai, Fei Zhao, Chengjian Jiang, Liping Meng, Yan Guo, Changzuan Zhou, Sunlei Pan, Hui Lin, Hangqi Luo, Feidan Gao, Tingjuan Ni, Jie Zhang, Na Lin, Wenqiang Lu, Chuanjing Zhang, Zhenzhu Sun, Xingxiao Huang, Jingfan Weng, Shimin Sun, Qi Yang, Shuqing Liu, Liuxu Yao, Jianyu Xia, Jinjin Yang, Ting Xu, Sihao Ju, Wenqing Xie, Nan Liu, Hanlin Zhang, Jing Sun, Jiaoying Song, Zhuonan Wu, Songqing Hu, Haowei Wu, Xiaomin Xu, Peipei Zhang, Zuoquan Zhong, Jiedong Zhou, Tingting Lv, Shijia Sun, Jinjin Hao, Hang Zhang, Yiping Yu, Jieting Zhang, Haijun Yu, Haifei Lou, Fang Wang, Ke Wang, Bingjie Zhao, Yefei Gao, Zeyu Shen, Hanxuan Liu, Tao Zhang, Juntao Yang, Wenwen Han, Zining Chen, Ying Zhu, Kaiyue Ma, Xiaofeng Zhao, Thapa Adesh Bahadur, Abdullahi Mohamud Hilowle, et al.